Anti Inflai for Beginners: 70+ Recipes For A Healthy You

☐ **Copyright 2017. All rights reserved.**

This document is geared towards providing exact and reliable information in regards to the topic and issue covered. The publication is sold with the idea that the publisher is not required to render accounting, officially permitted, or otherwise, qualified services. If advice is necessary, legal or professional, a practiced individual in the profession should be ordered.

- From a Declaration of Principles which was accepted and approved equally by a Committee of the American Bar Association and a Committee of Publishers and Associations.

In no way is it legal to reproduce, duplicate, or transmit any part of this document in either electronic means or in printed format. Recording of this publication is strictly prohibited and any storage of this document is not allowed unless with written permission from the publisher. All rights reserved.

The information provided herein is stated to be truthful and consistent, in that any liability, in terms of inattention or otherwise, by any usage or abuse of any policies, processes, or directions contained within is the solitary and utter responsibility of the recipient reader. Under no circumstances will any legal responsibility or blame be held against the publisher for any reparation, damages, or monetary loss due to the information herein, either directly or indirectly.

Respective authors own all copyrights not held by the publisher.

The information herein is offered for informational purposes solely, and is universal as so. The presentation of the information is without contract or any type of guarantee assurance.

The trademarks that are used are without any consent, and the publication of the trademark is without permission or backing by the trademark owner. All trademarks and brands within this book are for clarifying purposes only and are the owned by the owners themselves, not affiliated with this document.

Introduction:

What is Anti Inflammatory Diet

Inflammation is a response from your immune system to help heal your body. This can be useful when you have an injury or actual issue within your body. It increases white blood cell counts and gives the body the ability to protect organs and tissue from outside invaders. Inflammation is exactly what it sounds like. It is the swelling and redness of tissues, muscles, and other parts of your body.

The issue with inflammation is that it can be too active. It can work when and where it isn't supposed to. It can over-load our bodies, joints, organs, and lives with too much swelling. One of the most common examples of inflammation causing unnecessary swelling is arthritis. Your body isn't listening to you. You need to make it stop, and take control of your own inflammation.

Your body goes through a lot on a daily basis. It takes on and battles toxins, conquers stress, does everything you ask it to, digests everything you put in your mouth, and much more. The human body was not meant to conquer as many un-natural products as it does today. From smog to stress to processed foods, it's no wonder inflammation is a huge problem. Take on this anti inflammatory diet as a tool to help you change your life for the better.

Causes:

- Injury
- Infection

- Obesity/ Poor diet
- High Blood Sugar
- Oxidative Stress

Inflammation can be caused by a variety of different factors, including many lifestyle factors. It is important to enhance our immune system and strengthen our tissues as a protective mechanism against acute inflammation. Chronic inflammation can be helped by altering dietary choices as well as by taking dietary supplements.

Eating foods which are high in omega-6 fatty acids (arachadonic acid) like red meat, egg yolks, and other foods high in "bad fats" will contribute to amounts of inflammation in the body. Additionally, eating foods high in sugar will also contribute to inflammation through another mechanism. As our lives become increasingly stressful, and it becomes increasingly harder to find time or the resources to prepare healthy, well-rounded meals, our bodies are subject to more and more inflammation.

When we are stressed, our bodies release cortisol, which leads to a higher accumulation of fat in the body as well as a weakening of the immune system, leading to higher levels of inflammation. It is important to manage your emotional health and everyday stress levels in order to manage inflammation as well. Stress comes from a variety of different levels, and targeting stress can have a dramatic effect on various other areas of our bodies. You can read more about stress in our stress management protocol.

As the body seeks to repair this damage, it is important to determine what the causative factor was that led to the initial damage. Ask yourself, due to your lifestyle choices, is your inflammation related to any of the following probable causes?

Injury or Wounds: Damage to a tissue may result to inflammation as the body tries to draw circulation to the area as well as recruit other cells for help in order to repair the damage as quickly as possible.

Infection: Similar to the response when a tissue is injured, when a tissue (collection of cells) is invaded by a virus, bacteria or another pathogen, inflammation will result as a natural immune response in order to alleviate the infection as quickly as possible.

Obesity/ Poor diet: As we mentioned earlier, your ratio of fatty acids has a tremendous impact on the amount of inflammation in your body. You can control this ratio through your diet. Foods high in omega-6's (arachadonic acid) or "bad fats" contribute to inflammation. Additionally, eating foods high in sugar can lead to issues with inflammation as well.

High Blood Sugar: Having high blood sugar contributes to a process called glycation. When you have sustained high blood sugar levels, those sugar molecules attach to proteins and fats (where they shouldn't be!) disrupting and damaging tissues, resulting in the product known as AGE's (advanced glycation end products). These AGE's then bind to the cells, and cause higher amounts of inflammation. You can learn more about how to protect yourself in our high blood sugar protocol.

Oxidative Stress: Oxidative stress refers to the amount of free radicals occur throughout our bodies. Our mitochondria are the site of the most oxidative stress (as the site of energy production), and can become dysfunctional or start to degrade due to poor diet, smoking or other factors.

Symptoms:

For Acute inflammation only:

- Discomfort
- Heat
- Loss of function
- Redness
- Swelling

Note: Chronic Inflammation does not normally present itself with symptoms. It is important to perform the appropriate blood testing in order to protect yourself. You can learn more about blood testing here.

Table of Contents

The Complete Anti Inflammatory Diet for Beginners......1

Introduction:............................4

    What is Anti Inflammatory Diet..................4
    Causes:........................5
    Symptoms:.......................7

Chapter 1) The anti-inflammation diet...............................9

    Benefits of the anti-inflammation diet......................10
    The ideal nutritional balance....................11
    Foods to Avoid...........................12

Chapter 2) Breakfast Recipes:...............................15

    High Protein Breakfast Gold..................15
    Apple Breakfast Dream....................16
    Smooth Blueberries.....................18
    Spicy Scrambled Eggs......................19
    Avocado Smoothie..................20
    Breakfast Mexicana....................21
    Ultimate Skinny Granola................23
    Apple Chia Delight......................24
    Tasty Apple Almond Coconut Medley..................25
    Choco Nut Skinny Muesli Balls...............25

Chapter 3) Soups and Stews:...............................27

    Coconut Thai Soup.....................27
    Roasted Tasty Tomato Soup.......................28
    Thai Coconut Turkey Soup......................30
    Cheeky Chicken Soup....................31
    Triple Squash Delight Soup.....................32

Ginger Carrot Delight Soup......................33
Wonderful Watercress Soup..................35
Curried Butternut Soup........................37

Celery Cashew Cream Soup......................38

Chapter 4) Side Dishes:.................................39

Sweet Potatoes with Garlic......................39
Zucchini and Italian Spaghetti..................41
Wintry Weather Stir Fry........................42
Sweetie Skinny Crackers.............43
Sweet Melon.............44
Cinnamon Coconut Surprise......................46
Basil Pesto......................47

Chapter 5) Meat Recipes:................48

Turkey Eastern Surprise.................48
Roasted Lemon Herb Chicken....................49
Basil Turkey with Roasted Tomatoes.................50
Chicken & Broccoli........................51
Chili-Garlic Ostrich or Venison Skewers..............53
Creamy Chicken Casserole...............54
Spectacular Spaghetti and Delish Turkey Balls.....54
Sensational Courgette Pasta and Turkey Bolognaise......................56
Chicken Fennel Stir-Fry...........................57
Moroccan Madness.............................58

Chapter 6) Seafood:.......................................60

Sexy Shrimp with Delish Veggie Stir Fry...........60
Salmon Burgers......................61
Crab Salad......................62
Salmon & Salad......................63

Shrimp on Sticks......................64
Delicious Fish Stir Fry................................65
Delicious Salmon in Herb Crust....................66
Salmon Mustard Delish............................67

Chapter 7) Vegan Dishes :..68

Easy Pumpkin Chili...............................68
Simple Veggie Burger.............................69
Spectacular Spinach Brownies.........................70
Wintry Weather Stir Fry..............................71
Skinny Delicious Slaw...............................73
Cauliflower Couscous...............................74
Beetroot and blue cheese risotto........................75
Pristine Pumpkin Divine........................76
Eggplant Divine................................77
Raw Pineapple Coconut Vegan Cheesecake.........78

Chapter 8) Salads:..80

Coriander, Cumin and Chick Pea Salad................80
Mozzarella Salad with Heirloom, Grape or Cherry Tomatoes........................81
Chicken Basil Avo Salad..............................83

Turkey Taco Salad...............................85
Cheeky Turkey Salad.........................87
Macadamia Chicken Salad......................88
Rosy Chicken Supreme Salad........................89

Chapter 9) Dessert:..92

Sugar-Free Nut Cake...............................92
Ginger & Oats................................93
Sliced almonds with Apple Honey Mousse................94

Sesame & Almond Cakes.........................95
Chestnut-Cacao Cake....................96
Extra Dark Choco Delight.........................97
Nut Butter Truffles.................................98
Fetching Fudge..100
11) Conclusion..101

Chapter 1) The anti-inflammation diet

One of the most common complaints from patients suffering with inflammation is the debilitating discomfort they have to endure on a daily basis. I mean, going to bed after suffering from a painful bout of diarrhea/ constipation or abdominal cramps (the symptoms can be different for different people) while knowing fully well, that you're most likely to endure the same ordeal the next day too can be quite disheartening. While most people perceive prescription and anti-inflammatory drugs as the only solution, some others (the smart ones) explore lifestyle and dietary changes that when combined with medicine give them the results they're looking for. Having explored all of the above combinations, I recommend that you incorporate a balanced mix of the two. You see, while it's important that you continue your current course of medicine, it's equally important that you consume foods that aid better gut-health.

What you need is a complete diet plan that tells what food is good for you and what is not-like the anti-inflammation diet plan. The anti-inflammation diet is a little more than what is generally perceived as a diet. First off, the diet does not particularly target weight loss (although you can lose weight while on it), nor does it recommend you stay on it for a fixed period of time. On the contrary, the anti-inflammation diet has been specifically designed for one purpose-to reduce inflammation and suppress symptoms that are triggered by it.

Based on scientific knowledge, it tells you what foods to consume and what to avoid when you're trying to overcome chronic inflammation. It also shows you ways to select and prepare anti-inflammatory foods-foods that can help reduce inflammation and prevent it from flaring up again. Finally, it works around a holistic approach to give you all-round nutrition and energy. You see, when you are no longer eating foods that are known to cause inflammation, you give yourself a greater chance at fighting the illness and even reversing it sometimes.

Benefits of the anti-inflammation diet

In addition to suppressing symptoms of acute or chronic inflammation, the anti-inflammation diet has been scientifically designed to address and control a host of other secondary conditions that occur as an outcome of inflammation. The diet: **Lowers the risk of heart ailments and reduces bad cholesterol** Given that inflammation is most often the root cause of all other health problems, nipping it in the bud will help strengthen the gut and bounce off any secondary disease. Now, we already know how inflammation weakens the heart and causes heart-related problems. We also know how chronic inflammation can weaken the gut and allow harmful bacteria and bad cholesterol to reside in your body. As these levels of bad cholesterol and bacteria increase, they clog the arteries and prevent it from functioning properly, eventually leading to various heart-related problems. Consuming anti-inflammatory foods not only aid better digestion but also reduce the presence of parasites and bad cholesterol, which in turn lowers the risks of heart ailments.

Helps in weight loss While the anti-inflammation diet does not target drastic weight loss as its most important deliverable, the fact that you'll be eating only wholesome and healthy foods while on the diet infers that you're most likely to drop those extra kilos over a course of time.

Prevents and controls diabetes Several years ago, researches identified high levels of inflammation in the bodies of those suffering with type-2 diabetes. You see, as patients with diabetes do not produce enough insulin to regulate the amounts of sugar in their blood, they suffer a greater risk to problems such as obesity and inflammation-both of which are known contributors to type-2 diabetes.

Therefore, consuming a diet that prevents the trigger patterns of the disease can ultimately prevent type-2 diabetes too.

Reduces the risk of Cancer, Alzheimer's, and IBS
Prolonged inflammation can injure your body's healthy cells and weaken your immune system. Given that your immune system acts as the backbone for good health, a weak or overactive immune system can cause inflammation in various parts of the body and damage their functionality in the process. As organs become vulnerable to this attack, they become malfunctioned and in the process, lose their ability to deflect serious diseases such as Alzheimer's, Cancer and IBS.

Consuming anti-inflammatory foods will not only reduce inflammation and but also reduce the risk of any injuries to your immune system. With a healthy and functional immune system, you'll have the right tools to deflect IBS and battle even the most serious diseases, including Cancer and Alzheimer's.

The ideal nutritional balance

While we might have different dietary requirements (based on our age, gender and levels of activity), doctors recommend the following dietary strategies and nutritional balances for optimal health. Although it's not imperative that you hold this as a rule-book, it's recommended that you refer to it as a guideline while preparing your meals.

Estimated Caloric Intake
On an average, most adults are required to consume anywhere between 2,000 and 3,000 calories a day. While men and people who are particularly active require additional calories, women and individuals who are less active require fewer calories. Dieticians worldwide recommend that you consume 40-50% of your calories from carbohydrates, 30% from fat, and the remaining 20-30% from proteins. So as a thumb rule, it might help if you consume a small portion of the three foods in each meal. Additionally, a good tip to determine if you're

consuming the right amount of calories is to monitor your body weight. If you're consuming the right amount of calories for your activity level, then you should have no problem maintaining your ideal weight.

Foods to Avoid

In case you hadn't noticed, food is an important part of this diet. The anti inflammatory diet is about more than just counting calories and getting the right nutrients. Make sure you avoid the following foods, especially in excess. Some of them may seem harmless, but they are not taking care of your body like you need. They will cause more inflammation, pain, and digestion issues than they will solve.

Sugar – I know it can be hard to curve those sweet cravings, but it's important to avoid it, especially those processed sugars. Sugars and sweeteners can show up under all kinds of different names. Often, they are fall under names that end in "ose," like sucrose or dextrose.

Dairy – Milk is designed by nature to make baby cows gain weight. It makes it so they can grow up rapidly before they start feeding on their regular diet of grasses and natural foods. Dairy is extremely inflammatory and can wreck your diet and how you are feeling. In addition to this, the dairy that we consume every day is more processed which just continues to add inflammatory attributes and makes you feel even more miserable.

Gluten and Refined Breads – Gluten is a man-made substance that resides in almost every refined grain. It makes you feel worse and causes inflammation and irritation. This much processing is not what your body was made to digest. Gluten can be found in bread, pizza, pasta, and even cereal. This is one you want to be especially careful on.

Processed and Commercially-Fed Meats – When these animals are raised, they are kept in captivity, fed food that they aren't meant to eat, and kept alive with hormones and anti-biotics. When meats like pepperoni and sausage are processed, they continue to add ingredients that only cause you inflammation. Try and eat organic, grass-fed meats and stay away from anything that has extra processing.

Bad Oils – Vegetable oils, frying oils, hydrogenated oils, and partially hydrogenated oils all wreak havoc on your body. They cause inflammation on your body and will leave you feeling worse. If you have to use an oil for cooking, it is best to stick to olive or coconut oil.

Processed Foods – Processed foods, packaged foods, and fast foods can lead to large amounts of inflammation. These have items that are not naturally occurring and are meant to make you want to come back for more. Always look at the ingredient list and if it has something in it that you cannot pronounce or do not know what it is, stay away.

Alcohol – Alcohol, as fun as you may find it, dehydrates and inflames your body. They put a burden on the liver and put a high sugar content in your body. If you must drink while trying to control your inflammation, make sure you do so in moderation and with consideration to sugar and calorie content.

It's important that you pay close attention to your body and how different foods affect you. This list is by no means comprehensive. Different people respond to different foods in different ways. The best way to follow the anti inflammatory diet is to pay close attention to how you are feeling. Just like the beginning of the book suggests, write it down. Right down how you feel and what you eat. You may find that there are foods that are not on this list that end up making you feel worse instead of better. It is important that you take good care of yourself as you embark on this journey. Keep a running list of foods you know you should avoid. On that same token, don't be afraid to spoil yourself *in moderation*. If you are constantly stressed out and battling your cravings to an extent that prevents you from being happy, you will not take to this diet well. Find foods that make you happy and make you feel good. If you have to splurge, make it occasional and make it small. Stress only increases inflammation and prevents your body from focusing on what you need it to focus on.

Chapter 2) Breakfast Recipes:

High Protein Breakfast Gold

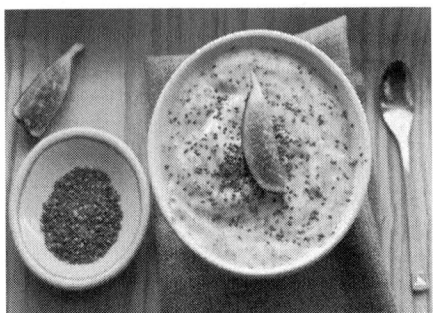

Ingredients:
1/2 cup (c). Flax-Meal, golden
1/2 c. Chia seed
Stevia liquid to taste
2 tbs. dark ground cinnamon
1 tbs. hemp protein powder
2 tbs. coconut oil, melted
1 tsp. vanilla extract

3/4 c. + 2 tbs. hot water

Instructions:
1. Begin to spread the dough out until its super thin, onto a parchment paper lined cookie sheet. Bake at 325 for 15 minutes, then drop it down to 300 and leave for 30 minutes.
2. Before dropping it, pull out the sheet and cut it. Put it back into the oven exactly like this, don't separate the pieces.
3. When the 30 minutes are up, pull it out and separate the pieces. Drop the pieces to 200 degrees F for 1 hour. They will be completely dried out at this point. Enjoy with almond or other nut milk!

Apple Breakfast Dream

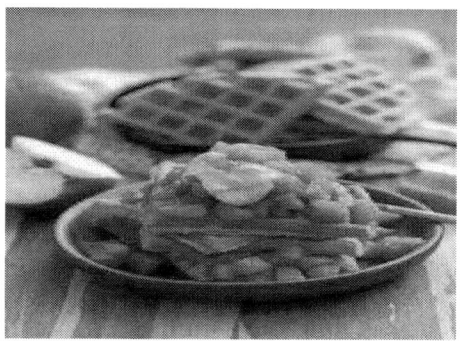

Ingredients:

2 Cup (C) raw walnuts

1 C raw macadamia nuts

2 apples, peeled and diced

1 Tbsp coconut oil

1 Tbsp ground cinnamon 2 C almond milk

1 14 oz can full fat coconut milk

Instructions:
1. Combine nuts and dates in a food processor until ground into a fine meal, about 1 minute; set aside.
2. Saute apples over medium heat in coconut oil until lightly browned, about 5 minutes.
3. Add nut mixture and cinnamon to apples and stir to incorporate, about 1 minute.
4. Reduce heat to low and add coconut and almond milk.

5. Stirring occasionally, let mixture cook uncovered until thickened, about 25 minutes.

Smooth Blueberries

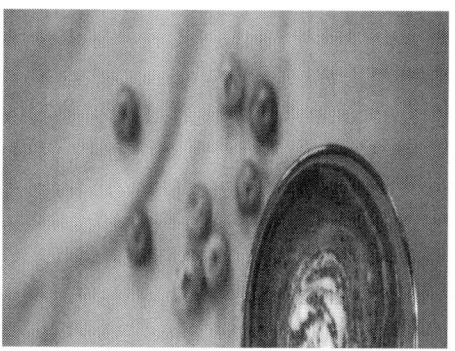

Ingredients:
- 1 Cup Blueberries, Fresh
- 1 Cup Greek Yogurt, Vanilla
- ¾ Cups Raspberries
- ¼ Cup Cranberries
- 10-12 Almonds, Raw
- 2 Tablespoons Coconut Milk

Instructions:
1. Mix everything together, and then just blend until it's smooth and ready to drink.

Spicy Scrambled Eggs

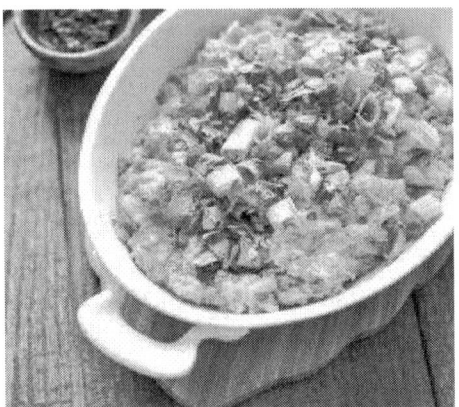

Ingredients:
1 tablespoon extra virgin olive oil

1 red onion, finely chopped

1 medium green pepper, cored, seeded, and finely chopped

1 chilli, seeded and cut into thin strips

3 ripe tomatoes, peeled, seeded, and chopped

Salt and freshly ground black pepper

4 large organic eggs

Instructions:
1. Heat the olive oil in a large, heavy, preferably nonstick skillet over medium heat.
2. Add the onion and cook until soft, 6 to 7 minutes.
3. Add the pepper and chilli and continue cooking until soft, another 4 to 5 minutes.

4 Add in the tomatoes, and salt and pepper to taste and cook uncovered, over low heat for 10 minutes.
5 Add the eggs, stirring them into the mixture to distribute.
6 Cover the skillet and cook until the eggs are set but still fluffy and tender, about 7 to 8 minutes. Divide between 4 plates and serve.

Avocado Smoothie

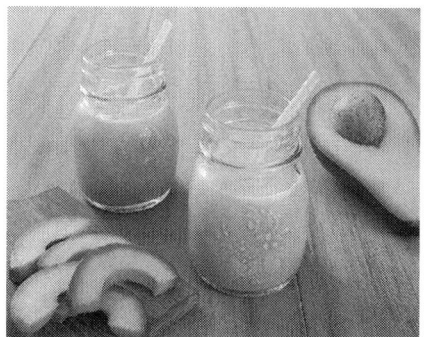

Ingredients:
1 chopped and peeled avocado
2 cups rice and almond milk, unsweetened

3 tablespoons honey

3 1 tablespoon lemon juice
4 5 ice cubes

Instructions:

Add all ingredients to blender then whirl until it is smooth.

Breakfast Mexicana

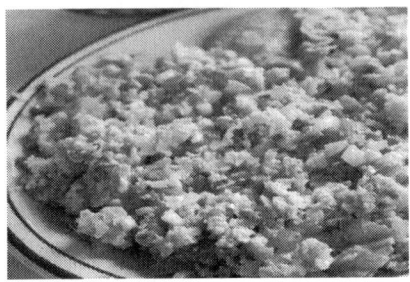

Ingredients:
For the tortillas:
2 eggs
2 egg whites
1/2 cup water
4 tsp ground flaxseed
Pinch of low sodium salt

For the filling:
1 avocado, diced
1/4 cup red bell pepper, finely diced
1/4 cup onion, finely diced
1/4 cup baked cod or other protein
Handful of spinach leaves
1 tsp coconut oil

Instructions:
1. In a small bowl, whisk together the ingredients for the tortilla. Preheat the oven
2. Heat a 10-inch nonstick skillet over medium heat and coat well with coconut oil spray.
3. Pour half of the tortilla mixture into the pan and swirl to evenly distribute.
4. Using a metal spatula, loosen the edges of the tortilla from the pan.

5. Cook a couple of minutes until golden brown on the bottom, and then carefully slide the spatula under the tortilla to loosen it from the bottom of the pan. Do not flip yet.
6. Place the pan under the broiler for 3-4 minutes until the tortilla gets a little bubbly.
7. Remove the tortilla from the pan, setting on a piece of aluminum foil. Repeat with other half of tortilla mixture.
8. After the tortillas are done broiling, preheat the oven to 400 degrees F. In a separate small pan, heat the coconut oil over medium heat.
9. Add the onions and peppers and sauté for 5-8 minutes, until soft. Add the spinach into the pan and wilt.
10. Place all of the fillings down the center of the tortillas and wrap tightly. Place into the oven for 5-8 minutes to set. It's so delish!

Ultimate Skinny Granola

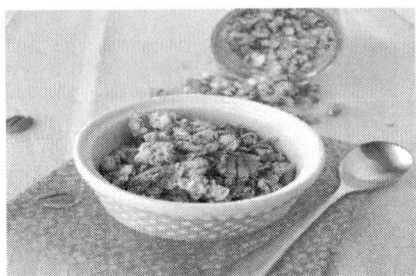

Ingredients:
1 cup of unsweetened coconut milk or unsweetened almond milk

Stevia liquid to taste

1 tablespoon each of unsalted ...
pecan pieces

walnut pieces

almonds
pistachios
raw pine nuts

raw sunflower/safflower seeds

raw pumpkin seeds

2 Tablespoons of frozen or fresh berry selection

Instructions:
1. Put all the nuts & seeds in a breakfast bowl.

add a teaspoon of pure liquid stevia and stir it well in.
2. Add the berries and milk.
3. If using frozen berries, wait for 2-3 minutes for them to get warmer.
4. The berries will now release some color into the milk, making it look really interesting. Enjoy!

Apple Chia Delight

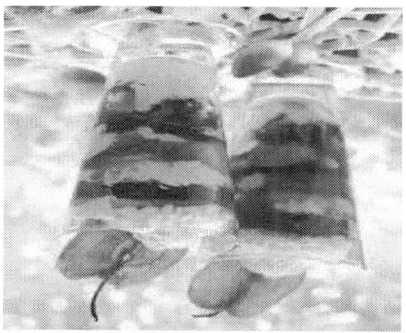

Ingredients:
2c organic chia seeds (black or white)
1c organic hemp hearts
1/2 chopped fresh apple
2tbsp real cinnamon
1 tsp low sodium salt
optional: 1/2c chopped nuts of your choice

Instructions:
Throw all of this together, mix it up, and enjoy with almond milk. Stevia to taste.

Tasty Apple Almond Coconut Medley

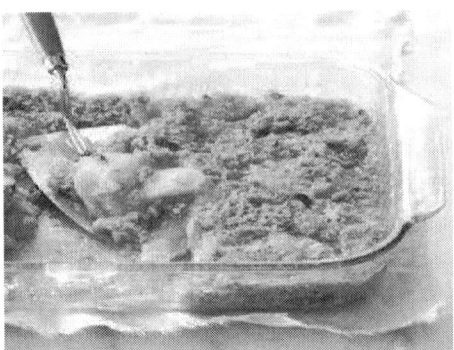

Ingredients:
one-half apple cored and roughly diced
handful of sliced almonds
handful of unsweetened coconut
generous dose of cinnamon
1 pinch of low sodium salt

Instructions:
1. Pulse in the food processor to desired consistency–smaller is better for the little ones! Serve with almond milk, or creamy coconut milk.

Choco Nut Skinny Muesli Balls

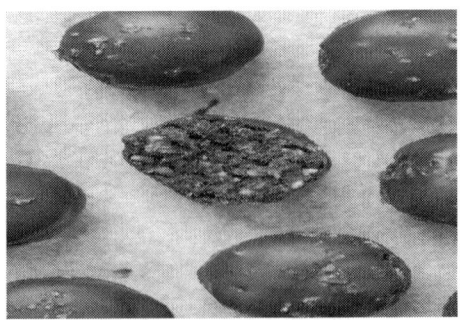

Ingredients:

1 cup of raw almonds
1 Tablespoon of coconut oil
¼ teaspoon low sodium salt
2 Tablespoon Coconut flour
1 egg white
2 Tablespoon plus 1 teaspoon of Cacao powder
pure liquid stevia to taste

Instructions:

1. First grind the almonds in a food processor or blender until you have a flour.
2. Add the ground almonds, low sodium salt, coconut flour, egg white, pure liquid stevia and cacao power to a bowl and mix with a spoon until you have a dough.

Either:

a) Place the dough onto a piece of parchment paper. Place a second piece of parchment paper over the top and roll it until it is ¼" thick. With a wet knife, score it into 1" squares. Place the parchment paper on a baking sheet when finished.

Or

b) Take a small pinch of the dough and roll into a ¼ round ball and set on a baking sheet lined with parchment paper.

3. Turn on your oven and set to 350 degrees and bake for 15 - 18 minutes for cereal balls or bake for 8 to 12 minutes for flat cereal.
4. Remove from the oven and let cool on the pan.
5. Top with your favorite nut or seed milk and enjoy

Chapter 3) Soups and Stews:

Coconut Thai Soup

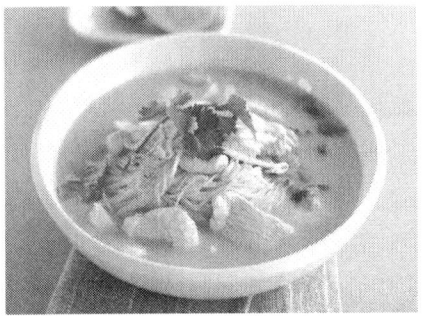

Ingredients:
- 5 Cups Vegetable Broth
- 2 Cans Coconut Milk
- Cup Shitake Mushrooms, Fresh & Sliced
- ¼ Cup Cilantro, Fresh & Chopped
- ¼ Teaspoon Red Pepper, crushed
- 3 Tablespoons Coconut Sugar
- 1 Tablespoon Olive Oil
- 1lb Cooked Shrimp, Chopped
- 3-4 Stalks Lemon Grass, Bruised
- 2½ Tablespoons Minced Ginger
- 2 Shallots, Chopped Fine

¼ Cup Lime Juice, Fresh

¼ Teaspoon Sea Salt, Fine

Instructions:
1. The broth and coconut milk should be mixed together in a large pan, heating it up over medium heat until it becomes warm.
2. Once it's warm, then add in all of your other ingredients, cooking for just a few minutes.
3. Stir in olive oil after you remove it from heat. Then, it's ready to serve.

Roasted Tasty Tomato Soup

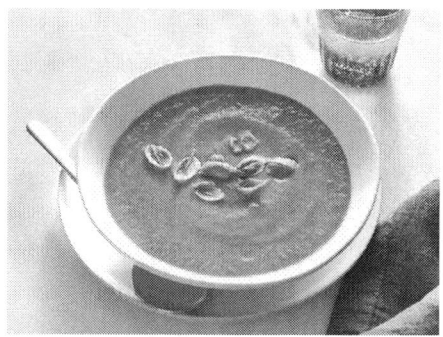

Ingredients:
1 lb fresh tomatoes
1 red onion, medium
1 small head garlic, pealed
1 tbsp olive oil
1 tsp low sodium salt
1/2 tsp fresh cracked black pepper
1 tsp oregano
3/4 cup low sodium chicken broth, homemade preferably
15 oz tomato sauce, canned - sugar and salt free
chives to top

Instructions:

1. Preheat oven to 375 degrees F.
2. Cube tomatoes and onion. Place on baking sheet. Drizzle with olive oil and sprinkle with seasonings. Slice butter into small pieces on top of vegetables. Roast for 30 minutes, stirring halfway after 15 minutes.
3. Allow roasted vegetables to cool for 10 minutes. Purée vegetables, broth and tomato sauce in blender until smooth, scraping down the sides several times while blending.
4. Heat tomato soup in a sauce pan allowing the soup to slowly simmer for a few minutes to blend the flavors together. Serve hot topped with chives.

Thai Coconut Turkey Soup

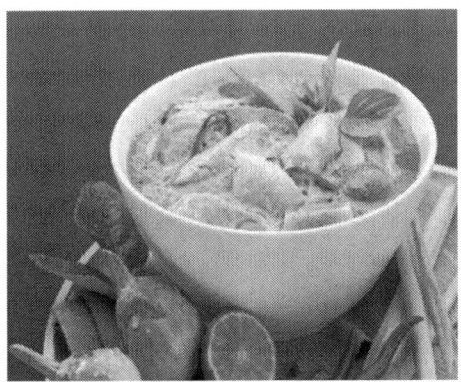

Ingredients:
A small splash of oil
1 onion, sliced thin
A big handful of shiitake mushrooms, cut in half
3 cloves of garlic, finely minced
1 inch piece of ginger, julienned

A handful of cherry tomatoes
4 cups turkey stock 1 cup shredded cooked turkey (or chicken) meat
½ cup canned coconut milk
low sodium salt to taste
A small handful of cilantro

Instructions:
1. Stir fry onion, garlic, ginger and the add mushrooms and tomatoes.
2. Add turkey meat and fry for a few minutes till slightly browned.
3. Add stock and simmer for 20 minutes.
4. Serve warm and sprinkle chives on top.

Cheeky Chicken Soup

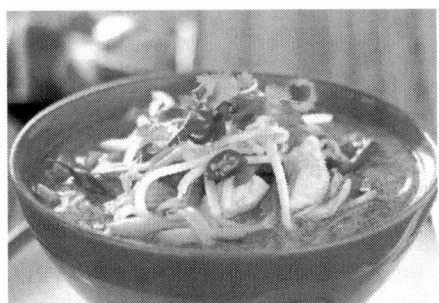

Ingredients:
2 large organic chicken breasts, skin removed and cut into ½ inch strips
1 28oz can of diced tomatoes
32 ounces low sodium organic chicken broth
1 sweet onion, diced
2 cups of shredded carrots
2 cups chopped celery
1 bunch of cilantro chopped fine
4 cloves of garlic, minced - I always use one of these
2 Tbs tomato paste
1 tsp chili powder
1 tsp cumin
low sodium salt & fresh cracked pepper to taste
olive oil
1-2 cups water

Instructions:
1In a crockpot place a dash of olive oil and about ¼ cup chicken broth. Add onions, garlic, jalapeno, low sodium salt and pepper and cook until soft, adding more broth as needed.

2. Then add all of your remaining ingredients and enough water to fill to the top of your pot. Cover and let cook on low for about 2 hrs, adjusting low sodium salt & pepper as needed.
3. Once the chicken is fully cooked, you should be able to shred it very easily. I simply used the back of a wooden spoon and pressed the cooked chicken against the side of the pot.
4. Top with avocado slices and fresh cilantro. Enjoy!

Triple Squash Delight Soup

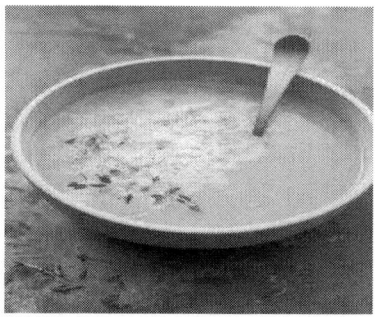

Ingredients:
1 butternut squash
1 gold acorn squash
1 white acorn squash
1-2 cups vegetable stock (depending on squash size, and how thick you want the soup)
2 cups diced turkey breast
1/4 cup light coconut milk
1 tbsp. olive oil
low sodium salt for seasoning

Instructions:
1Preheat the oven to 400 degrees.
2. Halve each squash, scoop out the seeds (and saving them for toasting), and then slice into 1-1 1/2 inch thick crescents.

3. Spread the squash on an aluminum foil-lined baking sheet and coat lightly with the olive oil. Season with low sodium salt. Roast for about 30 minutes, or until golden brown (turning once mid-way through baking).
4. When the squash has cooled from the oven slightly, spoon off the meat from the skin.
5. In a medium to large pot, bring the turkey meat, the meat of all the squash and 1 1/2 cups of vegetable stock to a boil. Turn the heat to low and stir in the coconut milk.
6. Remove from heat to puree the soup. You can use an immersion blender, or transfer everything to a traditional blender.
7. Blend until smooth, adding any additional stock to achieve the consistency you like.

Ginger Carrot Delight Soup

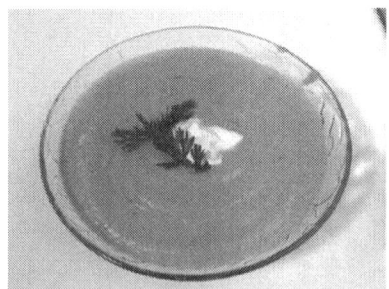

Ingredients:

3tbsp unsalted butter or coconut oil

1 1/2 pounds carrots (6-7 large carrots), sliced

2 cups chopped white or yellow onion 1 cup diced turkey breast

low sodium salt

2 teaspoons minced ginger

2 cups low sodium chicken stock

2 cups water

3 large strips of zest from an orange

Instructions:
1. Heat up the butter or coconut oil in a large soup pot.
2. Add the chopped carrots, turkey breast and onion to the pot and cook over medium heat for 5-10 minutes. Don't allow the carrots or onion to brown.
3. Add in the remaining ingredients (ginger, orange zest, water, and stock). The orange zest will be pulled out prior to puréeing so make sure they are in large, easy to identify strips rather than small pieces.
4. Bring to a boil then simmer for 10 minutes.
5. Remove orange zest strips.
6. Purée the mixture with an immersion blender. Or divide into 3-4 batches and blend in a regular blender.

7. I garnished my soup with a touch of olive oil and some freshly ground low sodium salt and pepper.

Wonderful Watercress Soup

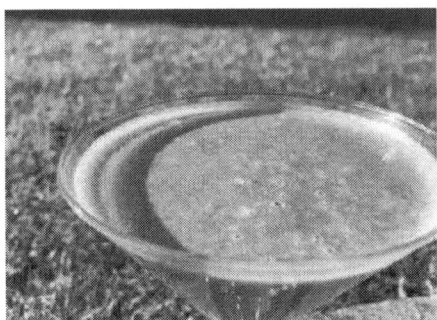

Ingredients:
1 quart low sodium chicken stock

1 medium leek

1 bunch water cress

1 large onion

1/2 celeriac root skinned and chopped 2 cups diced chicken breast - organic
low sodium salt and pepper to taste

Instructions:
1. Gently heat the chicken stock in the pot.
2. In the fry pan sauté the onion, leek and celeriac until soft.
3. Place the onion, leek, chicken and celeriac in the pot of stock reserving 1/3 aside.
4. Season with low sodium salt and pepper.

5 Add the bunch of watercress and simmer a few minutes until it is wilted.
6 With the immersion blender blend the soup.
7 Add the chopped vegetables that you reserved, back into the pot.

Curried Butternut Soup

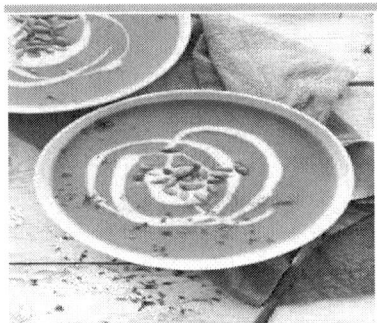

Ingredients:
2 medium butternut squash, cut in half lengthwise, seeds removed
(save for garnish)

1 cup diced chicken breast – organic
1 medium yellow onion, chopped

1 inch piece fresh ginger, peeled and diced or grated

1 tablespoon curry powder

1 can coconut milk (find BPA-free coconut milk)

1 1/2 C chicken broth

Coconut Oil

low sodium salt and pepper

Instructions:
1. Preheat oven to 425 degrees.
2. Melt a tablespoon of coconut oil in a roasting pan.
3. Place squash, cut side down in roasting pan.
4. Roast 45 minutes to an hour, or until fork tender.
5. Add ginger and curry powder and saute 2 more minutes.
6. Scoop flesh out of roasted squash and add to apple mixture. Stir to incorporate flavors.
7. Add coconut milk, chicken and chicken broth. Stir to incorporate ingredients and bring to a boil.
8. Simmer mixture, uncovered for 20 minutes.
9. Using either a high power mixer or an immersion blender, blend soup until it's smooth.

Celery Cashew Cream Soup

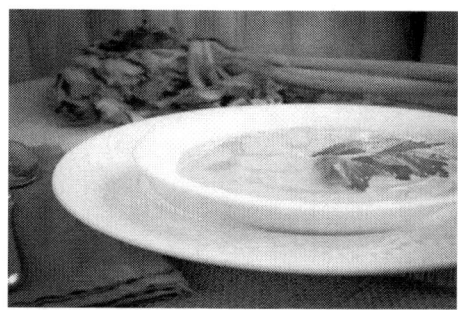

Ingredients:
300 grams celery, washed and chopped
1 small onion, chopped
1.5 tbsp olive oil
500 mls vegetable stock
40 grams cashew nuts
low sodium salt and pepper to taste

Instructions:

1. Heat the olive oil in a large saucepan then add the celery and onion, stir to coat with oil. Turn the heat low and put the lid on leaving the vegetables to sweat for 5 minutes.
2. Add the garlic, give a quick stir then add the vegetable stock and simmer for 10 minutes.
3. Add the cashew nuts to the saucepan and simmer for another 5 minutes or until the celery is cooked through.
4. Tip the soup mix into a blender and purée until smooth.
5. Season with the low sodium salt and pepper and serve.

Chapter 4) Side Dishes:

Sweet Potatoes with Garlic

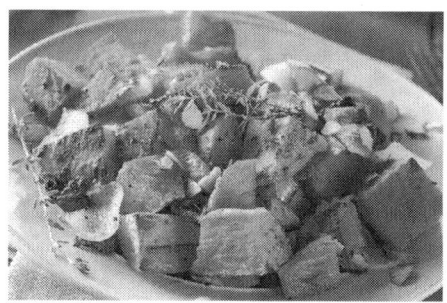

Ingredients:
- 5 minced garlic cloves
- large sweet potato (about 1 kg)
- ½ teaspoon of turmeric
- tablespoon of olive oil
- Fresh minced parsley

Instructions:
1. In large frying pan heat 1 tablespoon olive oil the sauté garlic until it becomes soft then set aside.
2. Saute turmeric and potatoes in olive oil until the potatoes are brown then add the garlic then sprinkle with parsley.

Zucchini and Italian Spaghetti

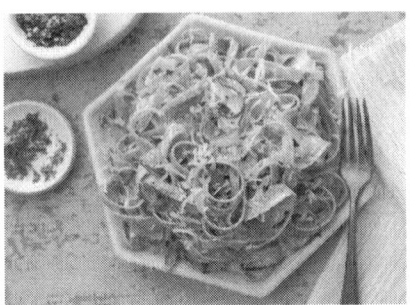

Ingredients:
- 24 oz. zucchini (thinly sliced)
- 1 oz. Spaghetti
- Pepper and salt
- ½ cup walnut oil
- 2 tablespoons of yeast flakes
- A few basil leaves

Instructions:
1. Heat oil in frying pan or skillet then add zucchini and garlic.
2. Turn up heat stirring often to cook through until crispy and golden outside. Cook and drain pasta then saute in a pan with yeast, basil and zucchini. Serve at once.

Wintry Weather Stir Fry

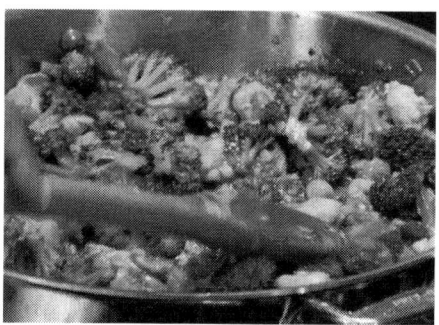

Ingredients:
1 broccoli (cut into pieces half inches thick)
2 baby bok choy (cut into small pieces)
2 carrots (cut in thin layers)
3 large sliced onions
Yellow or red bell pepper (cut into pieces half inches thick)
½ cup snow peas
1 minced cloves garlic
Light soy sauce or Tamari sauce
¼ cup olive oil
1 cup water
Brown rice

Instructions:
1. Add water to a large pan and bring to a boil. Add vegetables apart from the bok choy. Cover and let cook for approximately 7 minutes.
2. Drain then place back in the pan and put in bok choy. Mix oil, tamari and garlic then add to vegetables and cook for five minutes on low heat.

3. Add servings of brown rice (rice takes 40 minutes to cook on low heat).

Sweetie Skinny Crackers

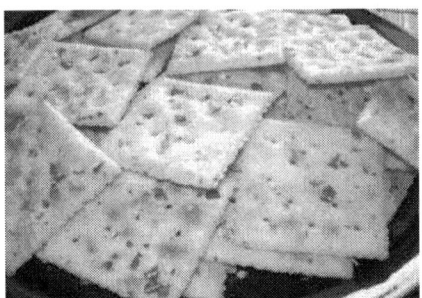

Ingredients:
1 egg

pure liquid stevia to taste

1 Tbspn coconut oil, melted

1.5 cups almond flour

.5 cup coconut flour 1 teaspoon cinnamon

Instructions:
1. Preheat oven to 350°
2. In a large bowl, whisk together the egg, pure liquid stevia and melted coconut oil Add the coconut and almond flour and stir to combine.
3. Give the dough a couple of kneads so it's well incorporated.
4. Turn the dough onto a piece of parchment paper and flatten a bit with your hands.
5. Place another piece of parchment on top and roll out with a rolling pin until it's about 1/8 inch thick.

6. Remove the top piece of parchment and cut the dough into 1/4 inch squares for cereal, and about 2"x3" for crackers
7. Sprinkle the cinnamon into the dough mixture.
8. Slide the dough with the bottom parchment paper onto a baking sheet and bake for 15 minutes.
9. Turn down the oven to 325° and bake for another 10-15 minutes, or until the cereal / crackers are crisp.

Sweet Melon

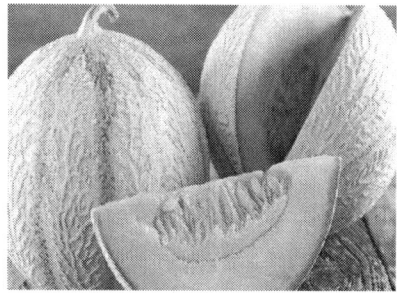

Ingredients
1/2 honeydew melon, cut into chunks (about 4 cups, or 1 1/2 lbs)
1/2 cup light coconut milk
1-2 leaves fresh mint (plus more for garnish)
1/2-1 tsp. fresh lime juice (or to taste)
1 cup ice
Drizzle of honey or coconut nectar, to taste (optional, depending on how sweet your melon is)

Directions
1. Cut your melon in half, remove the seeds, and slice away the outer rind.
2. Cut the melon into chunks, and add to your blender along with the coconut milk, mint, lime, and ice. Blend until smooth. Taste, and adjust sweetness with honey or coconut nectar.

3. Serve with a garnish of mint, or fresh melon slices.

Cinnamon Coconut Surprise

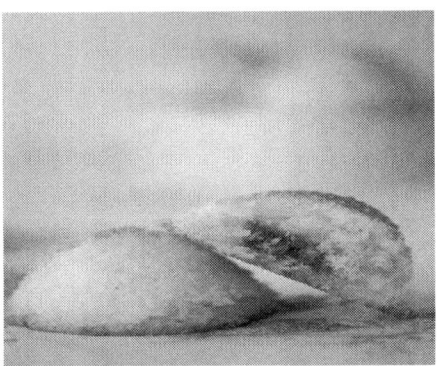

Ingredients
1/2 Cup Coconut Milk
4 Large Egg Yolks
1 Medium Banana
1/4 Cup Ice
1/2 tsp Cinnamon

Directions
1. Throw all of the ingredients into your high-speed blender and blast for 30 to 60 seconds until well combined.
2. Enjoy right away while still fresh, and give a little stir if separation occurs.

Basil Pesto

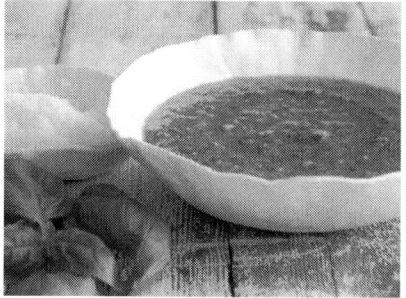

Ingredients
1 large bunch of basil (approx. 2 cups)
1/3 cup walnuts or pine nuts
2 medium garlic cloves, minced
1/2 cup Parmigiano Reggiano or other Parmesan cheese (optional)
approx. 1/3 cup extra virgin olive oil
salt and pepper to taste

Instructions
1. Place basil, nuts, garlic and cheese (optional) in food processor.
2. Run the food processor, pausing to add olive oil to reach desired consistency.
3. Salt and pepper to taste.

Chapter 5) Meat Recipes:

Turkey Eastern Surprise

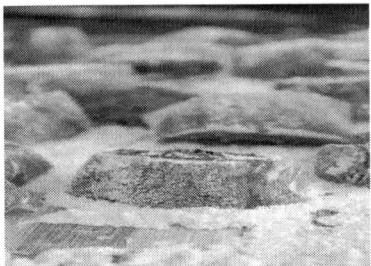

Ingredients:
For the salad:
2 cups grilled turkey, chopped
6 baby bok choy, grilled & chopped
2 green onions, chopped
1/4 cup cilantro, chopped
1 Tbl sesame seeds

For the dressing:
1 Tbl fresh ginger, chopped
2 Tbl coconut cream
1 Tbl fish sauce
1 Tbl sesame oil
2 Tbl fresh lime juice
1 tsp stevia powder or to taste

Instructions:
1. Combine all of the salad ingredients until well mixed.
2. Add all of the ingredients for the dressing into a blender or food processor, and blend until mostly smooth – there may be some small chunks of ginger left, that's ok.
3. Pour the dressing over the salad and toss lightly until coated.

4. Garnish with more sesame seeds if desired.
5. If possible let it sit for an hour in the fridge before serving so the flavors can really meld together.

Roasted Lemon Herb Chicken

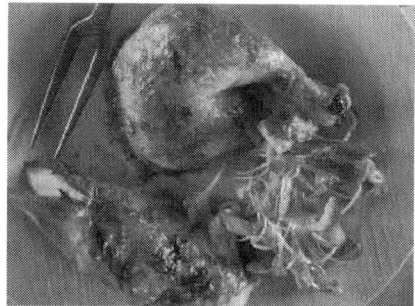

Ingredients:
12 total pieces bone-in chicken thighs and legs
1 medium onion, thinly sliced
1 tbsp dried rosemary
1 tsp dried thyme
1 lemon, sliced thin
1 orange, sliced thin

For the marinade:
5 tbsp extra virgin olive oil
6 cloves garlic, minced
Stevia to taste
Juice of 1 lemon
Juice of 1 orange
1 tbsp Italian seasoning – salt free
1 tsp onion powder
Dash of red pepper flakes
low sodium salt and freshly ground pepper, to taste

Instructions:
1. Whisk together all of the marinade ingredients in a small bowl. Place the chicken in a baking dish

(or a large Ziploc bag) and pour the marinade over it. Marinate for 3 hours to overnight.

2. Preheat the oven to 400 degrees F. Place the chicken in a baking dish and arrange with the onion, orange, and lemon slices.
3. Sprinkle with thyme, rosemary, low sodium salt and pepper. Cover with aluminum foil and bake for 30 minutes.
4. Remove the foil, baste the chicken, and bake for another 30 minutes uncovered, until the chicken is cooked through.

Basil Turkey with Roasted Tomatoes

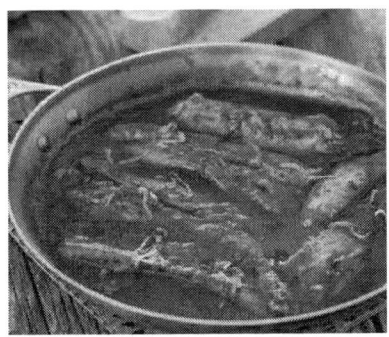

Ingredients:
2 turkey breasts
1 cup mushrooms, chopped
1/2 medium onion, chopped
1-2 tbsp extra virgin olive oil
Half cup thinly sliced fresh basil
low sodium salt and pepper, to taste
1 pint cherry tomatoes
Stevia to taste
Fresh parsley, for garnish

Instructions:

1. Preheat the oven to 400 degrees F. Place the tomatoes on a baking sheet and drizzle with olive oil and stevia. Sprinkle with low sodium salt and pepper and toss to coat evenly. Bake for 15-20 minutes until soft.
2. While the tomatoes are roasting, heat one tablespoon of olive oil in a large pan over low heat. Add the onions and mushrooms and cook for 10-12 minutes to soften and caramelize, stirring regularly. Clear a space for the chicken.
3. Season the turkey with low sodium salt and pepper and then place it in the pan. Simmer for 15 minutes or until the chicken is cooked through. Every 5 minutes or so, spoon the sauce in the pan over the turkey.
4. To assemble, divide the tomatoes between two plates. Place one turkey breast on each and then spoon the onions, mushrooms, and pan drippings over the turkey. Garnish with parsley.

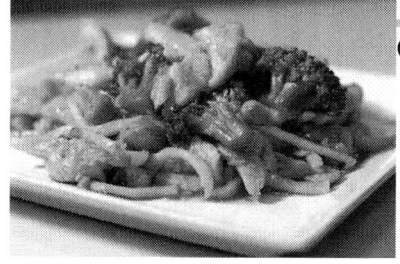

Chicken & Broccoli

Ingredients:
- 1 Teaspoons Olive Oil
- 1 Teaspoon Coconut Oil
- 3 Ounces Boneless Chicken Breast, Cut
- 2 Cups Broccoli, Chopped
- 1¼ Cups Snow Peas
- ¾ Cup Yellow Onion, Chopped & Peeled
- 1 Teaspoon Ginger Root, Grated
- ½ Cup Green or Red Grapes
- ¼ Cup Water

Instructions:
1. In a skillet, heat the oil over medium-highheat. Take your chicken, adding it, and sautéit until it's browned slightly. This can take from four to six minutes.
2. Add in your water, ginger, broccoli, onion, and snow peas. Stir often as you continue cooking until chicken is done and the water is reduced to a glaze. The vegetables should also be tender. This may take fifteen to twenty minutes.
3. Remember to add water when necessary.
4. The grapes are for a garnish to be added when you plate and serve the food.

Chili-Garlic Ostrich or Venison Skewers

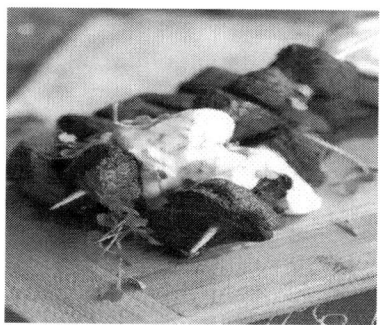

Ingredients:
6 Wooden Skewers, soaked in cold water for 30 minutes
2 Ostrich or Venison, diced
1 tbsp. Olive Oil
1 tsp. Red Chilies, seeds removed & finely chopped
4 Garlic Cloves, minced
6 tbsp. fresh lemon juice

Instructions:
1. Preheat oven to 350 F or preheat barbeque grill on high heat.
2. To make sauce, combine the oil, chilies, garlic, and lemon juice in a small bowl. Set aside for a few minutes.
3. Thread diced meat onto skewers and place on an oven tray lined with baking paper.
4. Pour chili and garlic sauce over the chicken, coating well.
5. Bake in the oven for 30-40 minutes or until chicken is cooked. If cooking on a grill, cook meat or poultry for 5-6 minutes on each side.
6. Eat with any of the delicious salad recipes.

Creamy Chicken Casserole

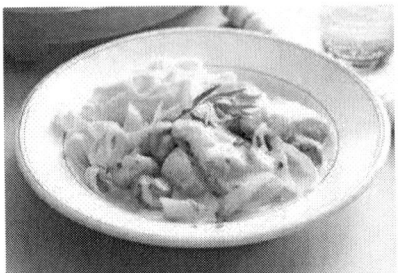

Ingredients:
2 cups cubed cooked chicken
1 1/2 cups cooked butternut squash
1/2 cup coconut cream,
1/4 cup coconut oil, melted
1 heaping cup green peas, fresh or frozen
1 tbsp apple cider vinegar
1/2 tsp low sodium salt
1/2 tsp oregano
1/2 tsp thyme
1 tbsp fresh parsley

Instructions:
1. In a large bowl, mash the butternut squash. Stir in the coconut cream, oil, vinegar, low sodium salt, oregano, and thyme.
2. Once everything is combined, add in chicken and peas.
3. Place the mixture into a large saucepan and cook over medium heat for 5-8 minutes.
4. Top with fresh parsley and serve warm.

Spectacular Spaghetti and Delish Turkey Balls

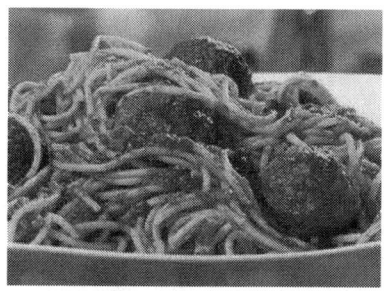

Ingredients:
1 spaghetti squash
Extra virgin olive oil,
low sodium salt and pepper
1 tsp dried or fresh oregano

For the sauce:
1 lb ground turkey
1 small onion, chopped
4 cloves garlic, minced
1 tbsp coconut oil
1 tomato, chopped
1/2 jar of tomato sauce
1 tbsp Italian seasoning
low sodium salt and pepper to taste
Fresh basil

Instructions:
1. Preheat oven to 400 degrees F. Using a sharp knife, cut the squash in half lengthwise. Scoop out the seeds and discard.
2. Place the halves with the cut side up on a rimmed baking sheet. Drizzle with olive oil and season with low sodium salt, pepper, and oregano. Roast the squash in the oven for 40-45 minutes, until you can poke the squash easily with a fork.

3. Let it cool until you can handle it safely. Then scrape the insides with a fork to shred the squash into strands.

4. Add chopped onion and garlic and cook for 4-5 minutes. Add ground turkey and brown the meat, stirring occasionally. Season with low sodium salt and pepper.
5. Add the chopped tomato, tomato sauce, and Italian seasoning and stir to combine.

Sensational Courgette Pasta and Turkey Bolognaise

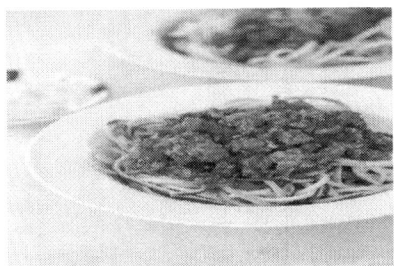

Ingredients:
4 medium zucchini

For the sauce:
1 lb ground turkey
1 small onion, chopped
4 cloves garlic, minced
1 tbsp coconut oil
1 tomato, chopped
1/2 jar of tomato sauce
1 tbsp Italian seasoning
low sodium salt and pepper to taste
Fresh basil, for garnish

Instructions:

1. Use a julienne peeler to slice the zucchini into noodles, stopping when you reach the seeds. Set aside.
2. If cooking zucchini noodles, simply add to a skillet and sauté over medium heat for 4-5 minutes.
3. Melt coconut oil in a large skillet over medium heat. Add chopped onion and garlic and cook for 4-5 minutes.
4. 4Add ground turkey and brown the meat, stirring occasionally. Season with low sodium salt and pepper.
5. Add the chopped tomato, tomato sauce, and Italian seasoning and stir to combine. Simmer on low heat, stirring occasionally.
6. Add the sauce to the noodles and ENJOY.

Chicken Fennel Stir-Fry

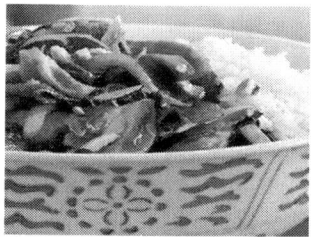

Ingredients:
3 chicken breasts or the meat from 1 whole roasted chicken
2 tablespoons coconut oil
1 onion
1 bulb of fennel
1 teaspoon each of low sodium salt, pepper, garlic powder and basil

Instructions:
1. Stovetop:

2. Cut the chicken into bite sized pieces. If chicken is raw, heat butter/coconut oil in large skillet or wok until melted.
3. Add chicken and cook on medium/high heat until chicken is cooked through. (If chicken is pre-cooked, cook the vegetables first then add chicken) While cooking, cut the onion into bite sized pieces (1/2 inch) and thinly slice the fennel bulb into thin slivers.
4. Add all to skillet or wok, add spices and continue sautéing until all are cooked through and fragrant.
5. This will take approximately 10-12 minutes.

Moroccan Madness

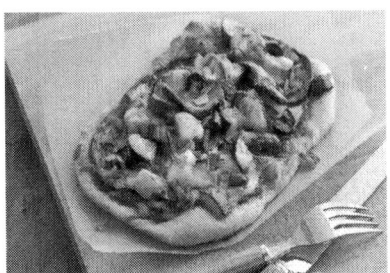

Ingredients:
1 chicken breast, chopped into pieces
1/2 tbsp olive oil
1/2 onion, chopped
1 bell pepper, chopped
1 cup diced courgette
2 cloves garlic, minced
1 tsp ginger, minced
1 tsp cumin
1 tsp turmeric
1/2 tsp paprika
1/2 tbsp oregano
1/2 can diced tomatoes

1/2 cup low sodium chicken stock
low sodium salt and pepper

Instructions:
1. In a pan cook the chicken in the olive oil
2. Once it's finished cooking, remove from pan and set aside
3. Add to the pan the bell pepper, onion, courgette, garlic, ginger and all spices, sauté until bell pepper and onion become soft
4. Add back in the chicken along with the diced tomatoes and chicken stock, let simmer for 10 minutes

Chapter 6) Seafood:

Sexy Shrimp with Delish Veggie Stir Fry

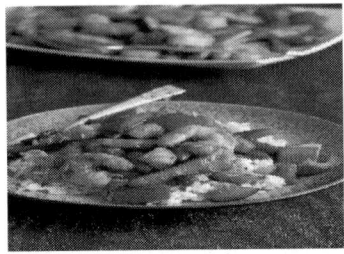

Ingredients:
1 1/2 pounds of shrimp
1 tsp. of coconut oil
1/2 cup of thinly sliced onion
1/2 red bell pepper. thinly sliced
1 cup of full fat coconut milk
2 tbsp. fish sauce
1 tbsp curry powder
2 tbsp. of chopped cilantro

Instructions:
1. In a large bowl mix fish sauce, garlic and ginger.
2. Heat the olive oil in a wok (or a large nonstick skillet) over medium-high heat.
3. Once it starts to shimmer add onion and chillies. Stir-fry the onions until they start to brown around the edges, about 2 minutes.
4. Stir in the bok choy stems and stir-fry for 1 minute.
5. Add the beaten eggs and cook until it's nearly cooked through about 2 minutes, stirring often.
6. Stir in bok choy greens, basil and lime juice. And stir-fry for 30 seconds or so, until the greens are wilted. Serve immediately.

Salmon Burgers

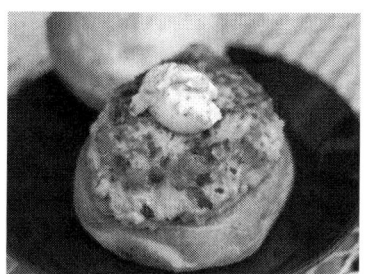

Ingredients:
- 1 14.75 oz. can of salmon (Wild Alaskan)
- 1 tablespoon peeled fresh ginger (finely grated)
- 3 minced scallions
- 1 tablespoon olive oil
- 1 large egg white
- 2 cups baby greens
- 1 tablespoon soy sauce

Instructions:
1. After draining the salmon add ginger and scallions and stir together in a ceramic bowl or large glass.
2. In a small bowl mix soy sauce and egg white then add to salmon mixture-make four patties from mixture (half inch thick)
3. Place twelve-inch skillet on medium flame and heat olive oil then put in patties and cook until golden brown on either side (6-7 minutes)

4. On each plate place half cup of greens then put the burgers on the greens and serve.

Crab Salad

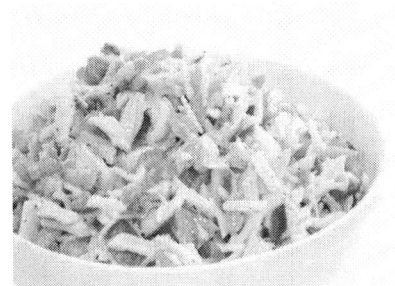

Ingredients:
- 5 servings:
- 2 tablespoons plain yogurt
- 1lb cooked crab meat
- ½ teaspoon salt
- 1 teaspoon lemon juice
- 5 heads Belgium endive, trimmed
- ¼ teaspoon cayenne pepper
- Chopped fresh chives

Instructions:
1. Cut the crab meat into chunks.
2. Take a bowl and combine the remaining ingredients. Afterward, add the crab meat and combine.

3. On the endive spears place the crabmeat and use fresh chives to garnish then serve.

Salmon & Salad

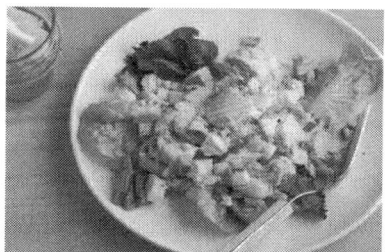

Ingredients:
- ½ cup Quinoa, Cooked
- ¼ Cup Pomegranate Arils
- 1 Small Avocado, Cubed
- 1 Cup Kale, Chopped
- ½ Cup Baby Spinach
- 3 Ounces-Wild Salmon, Boneless & Skinless

Instructions:
1. Make sure to season the salmon with salt and pepper, and then sauteit in a pan. It should be over medium to high heat, and you will want to pan sear it until it is a golden color.
2. If you like it medium rare, it should only be cooked for two to three minutes. Then, you'll want to set it aside as you prepare the salad.
3. Tenderize the kale, and then add in the spinach, stirring in the quinoa.
4. Drizzle with dressing as desired, tossing until it's combined. Top with the avocado and salmon. Sprinkle over the pomegranate arils.

Shrimp on Sticks

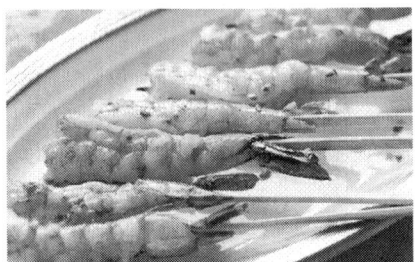

Ingredients:
1/2 lb shrimp, peeled and deveined

1/4 cup coconut milk

1 tsp fish sauce

6 gloves garlic, chopped

1/4 tsp each turmeric, cumin, low sodium salt

Instructions:
1. Heat olive oil in a large pan over medium heat. Add garlic and spices
2. Add shrimp and coconut last. Low sodium salt and pepper to taste and serve with a fresh squeeze of lemon.
3. Serve along side your choice of vegetable or fried cauliflower rice.

Delicious Fish Stir Fry

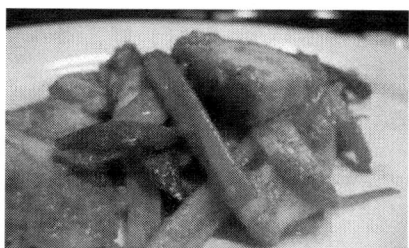

Ingredients:
200 grams any white fish fillet (cut into pieces)
1 Tablespoon Coconut or Apple ciderVinegar
1/2 Teaspoon Ginger and Garlic fresh pressed
1 small onion (quartered)
1/2 Cup Bell Peppers de-seeded and cubed (Red or Yellow).
1/2 Cup Mushrooms (any kind)
2 to 3 stalks of scallions (cut into 1.5 inch length)
low sodium salt to taste
1 Teaspoon Chili powder (Optional)
1 Teaspoon Fish Sauce – low salt
1/2 Tablespoon Extra Virgin Olive Oil

Instructions:
1. Put a pot with a bit of low sodium salt to boil and make sure your rice noodles are handy. Later, when the water has boiled, pop the noodles in and give it a stir.
2. Heat 2 tbsp. coconut oil in a wok or large pan.
3. Add the sliced garlic and grated ginger to the wok and stir-fry for 30 seconds.
4. Add the green onion and stir-fry 1 more minute.
5. Add the peppers and stir-fry about a minute. You want it just barely cooked, not limp and soggy.
6. Remove the vegetable mixture to a bowl and set aside.
7. Add another 2/3 tbsp. of coconut oil to the wok.

8. When the oil is very hot, add the green pepper and stir-fry for 1 minute.
9. Heat a ½ tbsp. of coconut oil, then add the pieces of fish and stir-fry. Stir-fry until just done and no more. To check, I like to cut open the biggest piece to make sure it isn't raw in the middle.

Delicious Salmon in Herb Crust

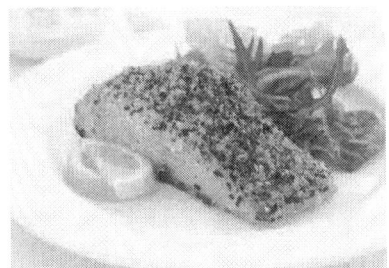

Ingredients:
2 salmon fillets (approx. 300g)
1 small onion, peeled and quartered
2 garlic cloves, peeled
1 sprig lemongrass, coarsely chopped
2 cm piece of ginger root, peeled
1 red chili pepper

Instructions:
1. Line a rimmed baking sheet with parchment paper and place salmon, skin side down, on the prepared baking sheet.
2. Generously season salmon with low sodium salt and pepper and top with sliced lemon and thyme.
3. Place baking sheet in a cold oven, then turn heat to 400 degrees F. Bake for 25 minutes.
4. Add lemon juice and serve immediately.

Salmon Mustard Delish

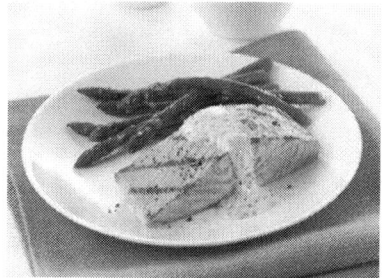

Ingredients:

5 tsp mustard seed

1/2 tsp garlic powder

1/4 tsp low sodium salt

1/4 tsp black pepper

1/4 tsp dried dill

1 1/2 lb salmon

Instructions:
1. Preheat oven to 200 degrees Celsius. (390 F)
2. Start by making the herb crust: combine the onion, garlic, lemongrass, ginger in the smallest bowl of a food processor
3. Process into a coarse paste.
4. Put the salmon fillets in an oven dish and spread the herb paste on top.
5. Bake for approx. 12-15 minutes until done, depending on the thickness of your fillets.
6. Serve with veggies of your choice and enjoy!

Chapter 7) Vegan Dishes :

Easy Pumpkin Chili

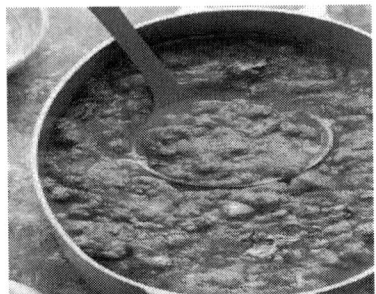

Ingredients:
- 1 Cup Pumpkin Puree
- 2½ Tablespoons Chili Powder
- ½ Teaspoon Sea Salt, Fine
- ½ Teaspoon Black Pepper
- 1 Tablespoon Cumin, Powder
- ½ Can Garbanzo Beans
- 15 Ounces Black Beans
- 1 Cup Vegetable Stock
- 5 Garlic Cloves, Minced
- 1 Large Onion, Sliced
- 1 Tablespoon Olive Oil
- 1 Cup Tomatoes, Canned

Instruction:
1. Take a large, clean pot and take the onion and garlic, mixing it with the olive oil to cook for about five minutes. It should turn soft, and it's best to cook over medium heat.
2. Take your canned tomatoes, pumpkin, black beans, garbanzo beans, and vegetable stock.

3. Add in half the chili powder and cumin. Add in all the salt and pepper, and then season more if needed.
4. Bring to a boil, and stir all ingredients together. Let it simmer for 20 minutes. Serve when cooled.

Simple Veggie Burger

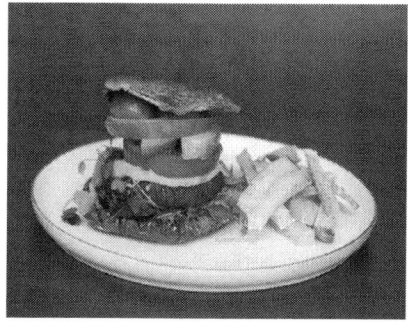

Ingredients:
- 2 cups fresh mushrooms (chopped)
- 1 cup cooked and drained beans (garbanzo)
- 1 clove minced garlic
- 1 medium chopped onion
- 2 eggs
- Fresh cilantro
- Cayenne pepper, salt
- ¼ cup Wheat germ (optional)

Instructions:
1. Warm a pan put in olive oil, then add onions and saute until tender (4 minutes).

2. Add garlic and mushrooms and cook for approximately five minutes.
3. In medium size bowl crush beans with a fork then put in the remainder of ingredients except the wheat germ.
4. combine everything and let stand.
5. Make burgers then roll wheat germ in and cook using a bit of olive oil for 3 minutes on each side.

Spectacular Spinach Brownies

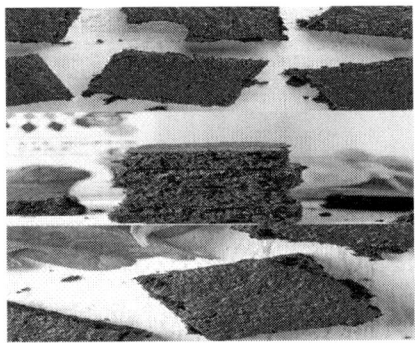

Ingredients:
frozen chopped spinach
sugar free chocolate
coconut oil
½ cup coconut oil
6 eggs
Stevia to taste
cocoa powder
1 Tspn vanilla pod
¼ tsp baking soda
½ tsp low sodium salt
½ tsp cream of tartar
pinch cinnamon

Instructions:
1. Preheat oven to 325F. Line a 9"x13" baking pan with wax paper or use a silicone baking pan.

2. Melt coconut oil and chocolate together over low heat on the stove top or medium power in the microwave. Add vanilla and stir to incorporate. Let cool.
3. Mix cocoa powder, baking soda, cream of tartar, low sodium salt and cinnamon.
4. Blend spinach, egg, together in a food processor or blender, until completely smooth (2-4 minutes).
5. Add coconut oil to food processor and process until full incorporated.
6. Add melted chocolate mixture and 3 or 4 drops stevia liquid to egg mixture slowly and processing/blending constantly.
7. Mix in dry ingredients and process/stir to fully incorporate.
8. Pour batter into prepared baking pan and spread out with a spatula.
9. Bake for 40 minutes. Cool completely in pan. Cut into squares. Enjoy

intry Weather Stir Fry

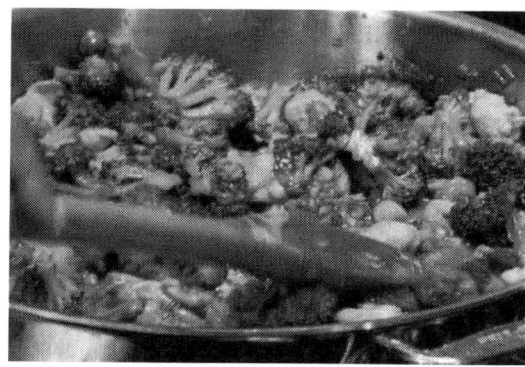

Ingredients:

- 1 broccoli (cut into pieces half inches thick)
- 2 baby bok choy (cut into small pieces)
- 2 carrots (cut in thin layers)
- 2 large sliced onions
- 1 Yellow or red bell pepper (cut into pieces half inches thick)
- ½ cup snow peas
- 2 minced cloves garlic
- Light soy sauce or Tamari sauce
- ¼ cup olive oil
- 1 cup water
- Brown rice

Instructions:
1. Add water to a large pan and bring to a boil.
2. Add vegetables apart from the bok choy.
3. Cover and let cook for approximately 7 minutes.
4. Drain then place back in the pan and put in bok choy.
5. Mix oil, tamari and garlic then add to vegetables and cook for five minutes on low heat.
6. Add servings of brown rice (rice takes 40 minutes to cook on low heat).

Skinny Delicious Slaw

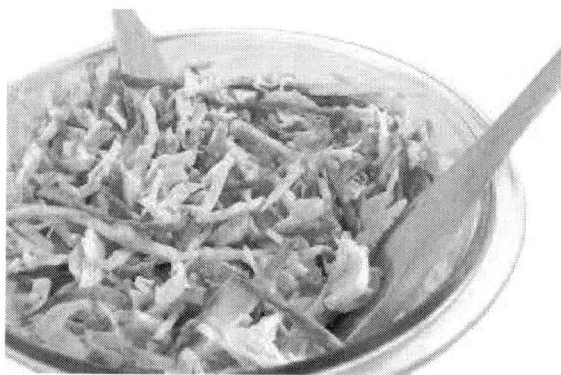

Ingredients:
1/2 head of cabbage (mix purple and white)
3 or 4 carrots
1 onion
3 tablespoons walnut oil
1 egg beaten
Stevia and low sdium salt to taste
1 Tbsp. fresh lemon juice
pepper to taste

Instructions:
1. Grate cabbage, carrots and onion and mix together.
2. Make dressing by mixing beaten egg, walnut oil, lemon juice, and seasonings.
3. Chill and serve.

Cauliflower Couscous

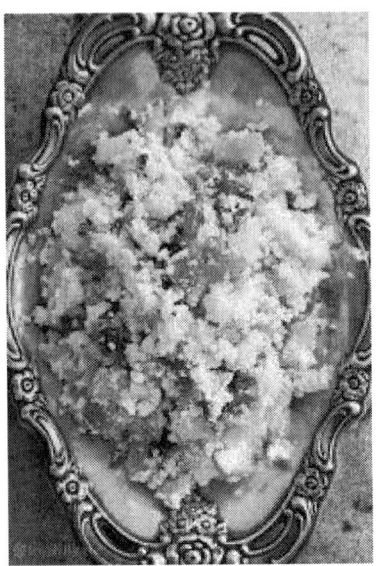

Ingredients:
1 1/2 Lbs cauliflower florets
1/2 cup parsley (VERY finely chopped)
1/2 cup fresh mint (very FINELY chopped)
1/2 cup chopped red onion
One cucumber finely cubed
4.5 to 5 Tbls fresh lime juice (about 2 fruits)
2 Tbls olive oil
1 teas low sodium salt
1 teas black pepper

Instructions:
1. In a food processor   pulse cauliflower until it looks like rice.
2. Put in serving bowl
3. blend the ingredients

Beetroot and blue cheese risotto

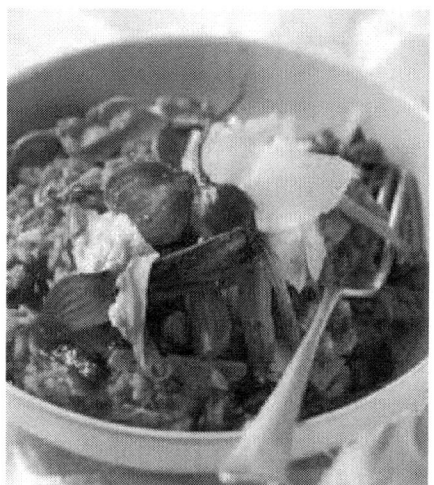

Ingredients

- 1 tbsp olive oil
- 1 cup chopped onion
- 2 cup chopped beetroot
- 200 g risotto
- Italian seasoning
- Salt and pepper
- Few sage leaves
- 2 litres of gluten-free vegetable stock
- 125 g of grated blue cheese

Instructions

1. Sauté onions and beetroot until cooked
2. Stir in the pasta and cook for 5 minutes
3. Add sage, seasoning, and stock and cook for 15 minutes
4. Stir in cheese, stir till melted and serve

Pristine Pumpkin Divine

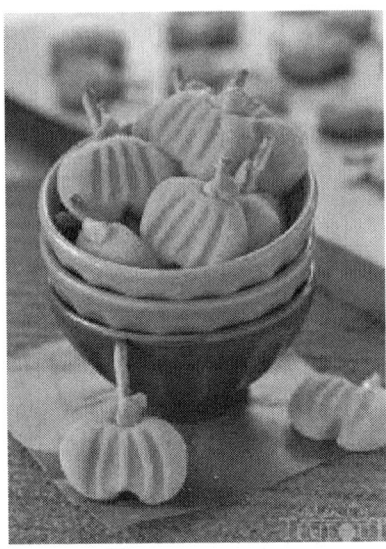

Ingredients:
2 cups blanched almond flour
½ cup flaxseed meal
2 teaspoons ground cinnamon (optional)
Stevia to taste
½ teaspoon low sodium salt
1 egg
1 cup pumpkin puree
1 tablespoon vanilla extract

Instructions:
1. Mix the ingredients.
2. In a separate bowl, whisk the egg, pumpkin and vanilla extract using a rubber spatula.
3. Gently mix dry and wet ingredients to form a batter being careful not to over mix or the batter will get oily and dense.
4. Spoon the batter onto a 9-inch pan lined with parchment paper or grease the pan bake at 350°F until a toothpick inserted into the center comes out clean, approximately 25 minutes.

Eggplant Divine

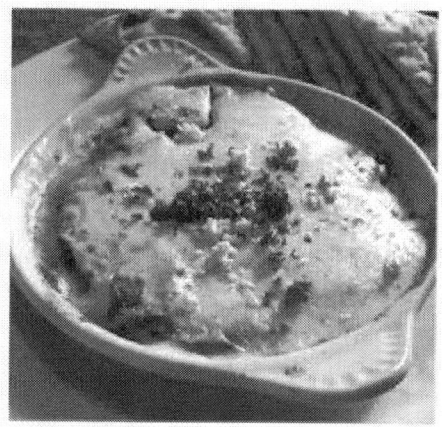

Ingredients:
1 large eggplant (about 1 pound)
1/2 cup olive oil
4 tablespoons balsamic vinegar
2 tablespoons pure liquid stevia
1/2 teaspoon paprika
low sodium salt

Instructions:
1. Wash eggplant and slice into thin strips. For ease in snacking you can cut long strips in half crosswise. Leave full-length for a more bacon-like appearance.
2. In a large bowl whisk together oil, vinegar, stevia, and paprika. Place strips in the mixture a few at a time, turning to make sure each is completely coated. If you run short of marinade, add a little more oil and stir it in with your hands.
3. Marinate 2 hours. Then, place strips on baking sheets

4. To dry in the oven: Line one or two rimmed baking sheets with parchment paper.
5. Lay strips on sheets, close together but not overlapping. Sprinkle on a little low sodium salt (you don't need much).
6. Place in oven on lowest setting
7. Check occasionally, and if any oil pools on the sheets, blot with a paper towel.

Raw Pineapple Coconut Vegan Cheesecake

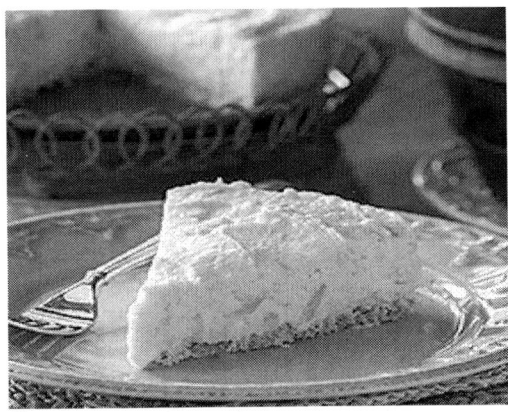

Crust:
   dates, soaked until very soft
   1 cup dried organic, unsweetened coconut
   Directions
   1. Place soften dates and coconut in food processor and process until well blended.
   2. Pat into the bottom of an oiled 7 1/2 inch spring form pan.

Filling:
   1/2 cups young Thai coconut flesh (about 5 young coconuts)
   1/4 cup coconut water
   1/3 cup nectar

coconut oil,
2 cups fresh pineapple

Directions
1. In high-speed blender, pureé the coconut flesh and coconut water together until smooth.
2. Add the agave, coconut oil. You want this to be quite smooth so blend away until it is.
3. Add 1 cup of the pineapple chunks.
4. Blend until incorporated.Pulse the remaining pineapple chunks in the food processor until well chopped.
5. Drain.Stir the pineapple into the coconut mixture, pour over crust and let set up in the refrigerator for 4 hours.
6. Move to freezer and leave until firm.

Chapter 8) Salads:

Coriander, Cumin and Chick Pea Salad

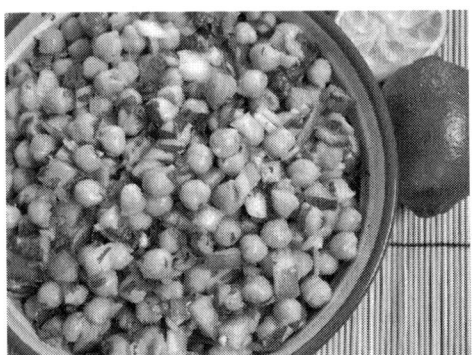

Ingredients: *Dressing:*
- 2 tablespoons white-wine vinegar
- 3 tablespoons fresh lemon juice
- 1½ teaspoons peeled and grated fresh ginger root
- 2 garlic minced cloves (mashed with ¼ teaspoon salt)
- ¼ teaspoon dried hot red pepper flakes (add more if needed)
- 1 teaspoon ground cumin (add more if needed)
- Black pepper (freshly ground)
- ½ cup extra virgin olive oil

Salad:
- 1 small bunch of thinly sliced scallions
- 2 finely chopped yellow or red bell peppers

- 4 cans chickpeas (19-ounce) - rinse and drain well
- Large Romaine Lettuce leaves
- ½cup fresh coriander (finely chopped)–add more if needed
- Lemon wedges

Instructions:

Dressing:

1. Whisk freshly ground black pepper, sea salt, cayenne, cumin, ginger root, garlic paste, and the vinegar and lemon juice in a bowl.
2. Start adding oil while whisking and keep on doing that to get it emulsified.
3. Taste and make adjustments if necessary.

Salad:

In a bowl combine coriander, scallions, bell peppers and chickpeas as well as the dressing then cover and let chill overnight.

Mozzarella Salad with Heirloom, Grape or Cherry Tomatoes

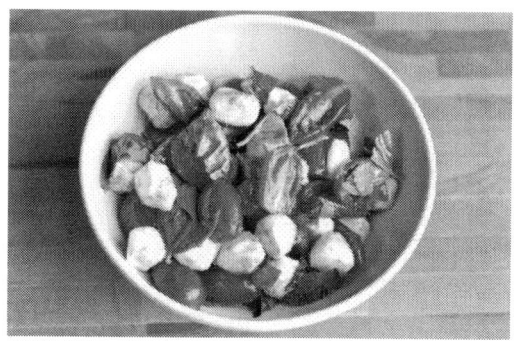

Ingredients: *Dressing:*
- Freshly ground pepper
- Sea salt
- 1 clove pressed or minced garlic
- 1 tsp. oregano
- 2 tbsp. fresh chopped basil
- 4 tbsp. Organic Extra Virgin Olive Oil
- 1 tbsp. Balsamic Vinegar

Salad:
- 8 oz. fresh mozzarella
- 4 to 6 large heirloom, on-the-vine or organic or tomatoes

Instructions:
Dressing:
1. Combine all the ingredients. Set aside.

Salad:
1. Tomatoes should be sliced to be half an inch thick.
2. If grape or cherry tomatoes are used do not slice them.
3. Cut mozzarella into eight slices.
4. Another option is to layer mozzarella and tomatoes. Use vinaigrette to drizzle over salad then season with pepper and salt and use fresh basil to garnish.

Chicken Basil Avo Salad

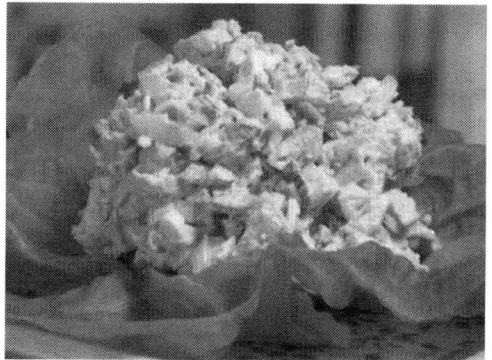

Ingredients:

2 boneless, skinless chicken breasts (organic, cooked and shredded)

1/2 cup fresh basil leaves, stems removed 1 cup sliced cherry tomatoes

2 small or 1 large ripe avocado, pits and skin removed

2 Tbsp. extra virgin olive oil

1/2 tsp. low sodium salt (or more to taste)

1/8 tsp. ground black pepper (or more to taste)

Instructions:

1. Place the cooked shredded chicken in a medium sized mixing bowl.
2. Place the basil, avocado, olive oil, low sodium salt and ground black pepper in a food processor and blend until smooth. You may need to scrape the sides a couple times to incorporate.

3. Pour the avocado and basil mixture into the mixing bowl with the shredded chicken and tomatoes and toss well to coat.
4. Taste and add additional low sodium salt and ground black pepper if desired. Keep in the fridge until ready to serve.

Skinny Chicken salad

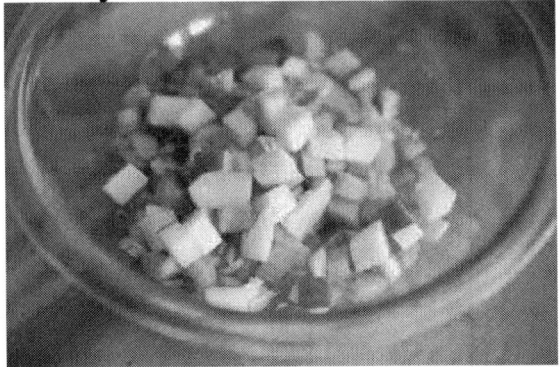

Ingredients:
Salad:
1 small cabbage
–
carrot

1/4 cup fresh cilantro, chopped

1/4 cup fresh mint, chopped

2 cups cooked organic chicken
Vinaigrette:
2 tablespoons coconut or rice vinegar
3 tablespoons sesame oil

juice of 1/2 a lime

1 chipotle pepper - optional 1 clove garlic, crushed

1 teaspoon fresh ginger, grated

Instructions:
Salad

1. Combine cabbage, carrots, scallions and radishes.
2. Top with chicken, cilantro and mint and set aside.

Vinaigrette

1. Combine the vinaigrette ingredients.
2. Taste to see if it needs any adjustments. If it is too spicy, you can add more lime juice to counteract it.
3. Drizzle salad with vinaigrette & enjoy.

Turkey Taco Salad

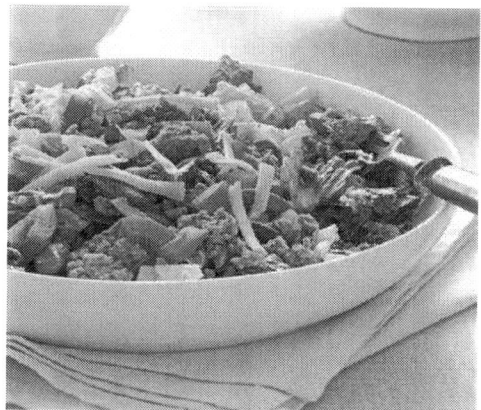

Ingredients:
1/2 lbs (ish) leftover turkey, cooked and chopped
taco seasoning

1 tblsp. coconut
1 tblsp rice vinegar
lettuce

Optional Toppings - sliced olives, tomatoes, red onion, avocado, bell peppers,
crushed sweet potato chips

Taco Seasoning:

Mix together,
- 4 Tbsp. chili powder,
- 1 tsp each garlic powder, onion powder, and oregano,
- 3 tsp each paprika and cumin,
- 4 tsp low sodium salt, and 1/8-1/4 tsp red pepper flakes.

Instructions:

1. In a skillet, heat 1 teaspoon oil and add in chicken - I like to fry it for a minute to give some extra flavor. Add in water and taco seasoning, let simmer until liquid is gone.
2. Meanwhile, shred, chop, and dice all your toppings.
3. Assemble, lettuce, optional toppings, chicken, leftover oil and vinegar dressing, and crushed chips.

Cheeky Turkey Salad

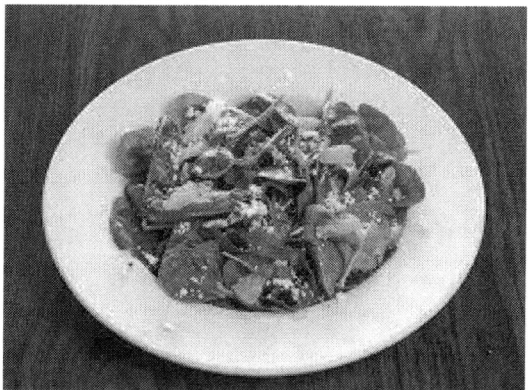

Ingredients:
For the Turkey:
1 lb boneless turkey breasts
1 tbsp olive oil
low sodium salt and pepper, to taste

For the Salsa:
1 large tomato, quartered
1/2 red onion, cut into large chunks
1 garlic clove, peeled

1 small bunch of cilantro leaves
Juice of 1 lime
low sodium salt and pepper, to taste

Instructions:
1. Preheat oven to 375 F.
2. Bake turkey breasts dipped in olive oil on a baking sheet for 35 to 40 minutes, until no longer pink in the center.
3. While baking, add all salsa ingredients to a food processor and pulse using the chopping blade until finely chopped. Transfer the salsa to a large bowl and clean out the food processor. You will be using it to shred the turkey.

(If you don't have a food processor, just dice the tomato, onion, pepper, cilantro and garlic and add to a bowl with the lime juice, low sodium salt and pepper).

4. Remove turkey from the oven and allow to cool. Once cool enough to handle, cut each breast into three or four smaller pieces and add to the food processor.
5. Pulse using the chopping blade until shredded.
6. Add turkey to bowl with salsa and mix well with a fork.
7. Refrigerate for at least two hours until turkey salad is chilled.

Macadamia Chicken Salad

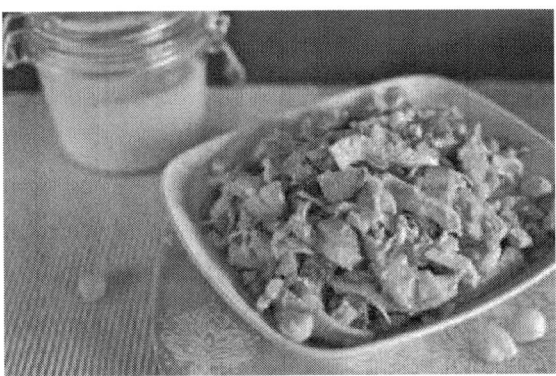

Ingredients:
1lb organic chicken breast
1tsp macadamia nut oil, or oil of choice
few pinches of low sodium salt and pepper
1/2 cup macadamia nuts, chopped
1/2 cup diced celery
2 tbsp julienned basil
1 tablespoon olive oil and 2 teaspoons rice vinegar
1 tbsp lemon juice

Instructions:

1. Preheat oven to 350.
2. Place chicken breasts on sheet tray, drizzle will oil and a pinch of low sodium salt and pepper.
3. Bake for about 35 minutes until cooked through.
4. Remove from oven and let cool.
5. In a large bowl shred chicken. Add nuts, celery, basil, dressing, and a pinch of low sodium salt and pepper.
6. Gently stir until combined. Eat!

Rosy Chicken Supreme Salad

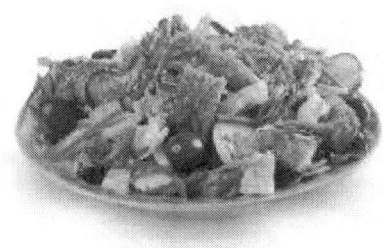

Ingredients:
For the chicken:
450g chicken mince, free range of course
1 long red chili, finely chopped with the seeds
2 garlic cloves, finely chopped
Little nob of fresh ginger, peeled and finely chopped
1 stem lemon grass, pale section only, finely chopped
1/2 bunch of coriander stems washed and finely chopped (I don't waste anything,
   save the leaves for the salad)
2 1/2 tbsp fish sauce
1/2 lime rind grated
1/2 lime, juiced

A pinch of low sodium salt
Coconut oil for frying (about 3 tablespoons)

For the salad:
1/4 red cabbage, thinly sliced
1 large carrot, peeled and grated
1/2 Spanish onion, thinly sliced
2 tbsp green spring onion, chopped
1/2 bunch of fresh coriander leaves (saved from the stems used in the chicken)
A handful of fresh mint or Thai basil if available
1/2 cup crashed roasted cashews or some sesame seeds

For the dressing:
2 tbsp olive oil
3 tbsp lime juice
1 tbsp fish sauce
1 small red chili, finely chopped

Instructions:
1. Once you've prepared all your ingredients for the chicken, heat 1 tbsp of coconut oil in a large frying pan or a wok to high.
2. Throw in lemongrass, chili, garlic, coriander stems and ginger and stir fry for about a minute until fragrant.
3. Add chicken mince and lime zest. Stir and break apart the mince with a wooden mixing spoon until separated into small chunks (this might take a while as chicken mince is quite sticky).
4. The meat will now be changing to white colour.
5. Add fish sauce and lime juice. Stir through and cook for a further few minutes. Total cooking time for the chicken should be about 10 minutes.

6. Prepare the salad base by mixing together sliced red cabbage, onion grated carrot, and fresh herbs.
7. Mix all dressing ingredients and toss through the salad.

Chapter 9) Dessert:

Sugar-Free Nut Cake

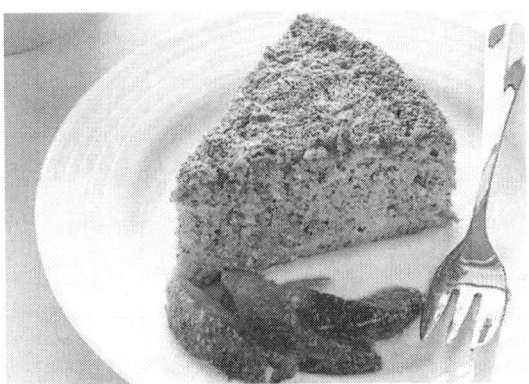

Ingredients: *Dry ingredients:*
- 1 tbsp oats
- 5 tsp baking powder
- 2 cups brown rice flour
- ½ teaspoon sea salt

Seeds: a mix of flax, pumpkin, sunflower and sesame seeds.

Liquid:
- 2 Eggs
- ¼ cup water
- 2 tbsp olive oil
- Tahini (optional)

To place on top of each nut cake:

- Herbes de Provence or other dried herbs
- Coarse sea salt
- 1 raw walnut (or almond) on each cake

Instructions:
1. Mix the dry ingredients then add the olive oil, eggs and tahini. Add water until a smooth dough is acquired (it should be sticky) so do not knead the dough a lot.
2. Make small buns and put them on greased baking pan. Put walnut or almond on top then sprinkle with coarse sea salt and herbs de Provence.
3. Place in oven and bake at three hundred and sixty degrees.
4. Fahrenheit for approximately half an hour. To ensure it is well-baked use knife to test bun.

Ginger & Oats

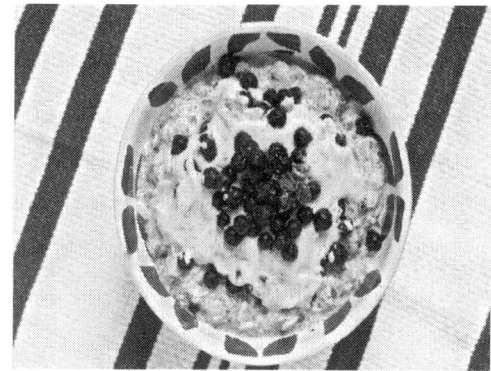

Ingredients:

- ½ Cup Oatmeal
- ½ Cup Water
- ½ Cup Coconut Milk
- 1 Teaspoon Coconut Oil
- ½ Cup Banana, Chopped
- 1½ Teaspoon Ginger Powder
- 1/3 Cup Fresh Blueberries

Instructions:
1. Everything except the banana should go into a pot to cook.
2. Cook until ready like you would for normal oatmeal, and then take it out and place into a clean bowl.
3. Add in the bananas, and eat while warm. If you do need something to sweeten it with, do not use sugar. A teaspoon of raw, local honey is usually best. Remember that the darker the honey the more taste and flavor it'll have.

Sliced almonds with Apple Honey Mousse

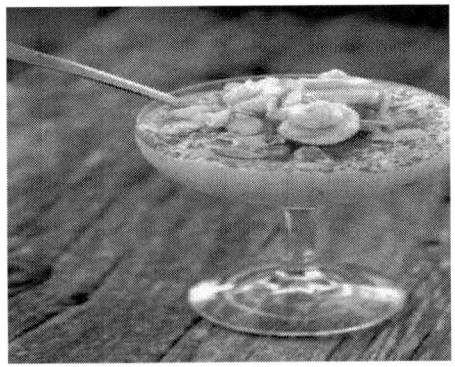

Ingredients:
- 2 tbsp honey

- 500 gr. apples (organic like Mutsu, Yellow Delicious, Winesap, Gala or Red Delicious)
- 2gr agar agar
- ½cup yogurt

Instructions:
1. Wash the apples the peel and chop them.
2. In the bottom of a large pot put in one-inch water then add agar agar, honey and apples and cover pot then turn the heat up. When it comes to a boil turn heat down and cook until apples are soft.
3. Stir apples until they are all crushed up or put in food processor and make a puree. Allow to cool.
4. Whip yogurt then add it to the applesauce. Pour into cups then place in refrigerator. Add honey and sliced almonds before serving.

Sesame & Almond Cakes

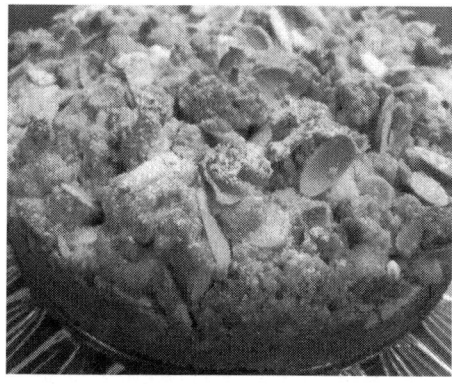

Ingredients:
- 200 g almond powder

- 3 Eggs
- 120 g brown sugar
- 40 g Tahini (rice flour can be used as substitute)
- 2 tsp orange or almond extract
- 3 tsp sesame seeds

Instructions:
1. Preheat oven to 200 degrees Fahrenheit.
2. Mix eggs, extract, tahini and sugar then put in almond powder and combine well.
3. Use sesame seeds to sprinkle then cook for approximately forty-five minutes.

Chestnut-Cacao Cake

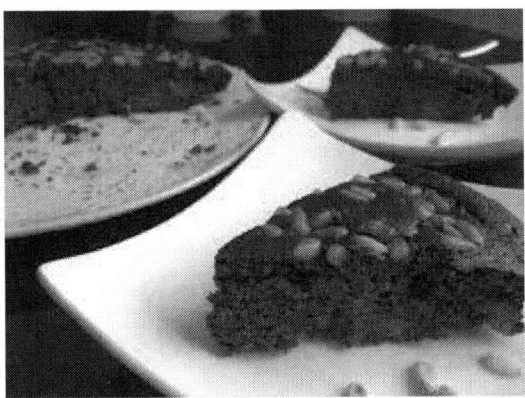

Ingredients:
100g (1 cup + 1 heaping tablespoon) chestnut flour
50g (1/2 cup) ground almonds (almond flour)
3 eggs, separate
1/2 teaspoon cream of tartar
35g (1/2 cup) raw cacao powder
Stevia to taste
3/4 cup coconut milk
1/2 teaspoon baking soda
Crushed chesnuts

Instructions:
1. Preheat oven to 180C fan (350F).
2. Grease a pie/tart pan.
3. In a clean mixing bowl, beat the egg whites and cream of tartar until stiff peaks form. Set aside.
4. In another mixing bowl, cream the egg yolks, chestnut flour, ground almonds, stevia, raw cacao, baking soda and coconut milk.
5. Fold in the egg whites and blend until the white is no longer showing.
6. Pour into the pie/tart mold.
7. Sprinkle with crushed chestnuts, if desired.
8. Bake for 35-40 minutes on the middle rack.

Extra Dark Choco Delight

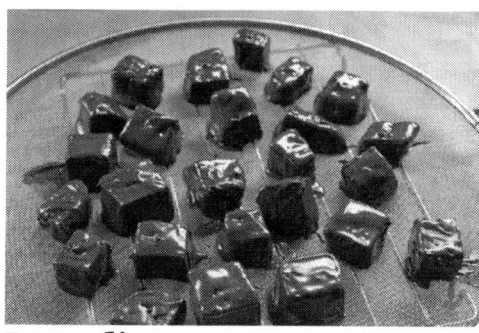

Ingredients:
1 egg
½ very ripe avocado
¼ cup full fat canned coconut milk
2 tbsp cacao powder
1 tbsp carob powder
pinch low sodium salt
pinch cinnamon
1 scoop vanilla flavored hemp protein powder
10g raw hazelnuts
2 tbsp unsweetened shredded coconut

Stevia to taste

Instructions:
1. Add the egg, avocado and coconut milk to a small food processor and process until very smooth and process until very smooth and creamy.
2. Add cacao powder, carob powder, low sodium salt, cinnamon and protein powder and process again until well combined and creamy.
3. Add hazelnuts and shredded coconut and give a few extra spins until the hazelnuts are reduced to tiny little pieces.
4. Serve immediately or refrigerate until ready to serve.
5. Garnish with a little dollop of coconut cream and cacao nibs or shredded coconut and crushed hazelnuts.
6. This will keep in the refrigerator for a few days in an airtight container.

Nut Butter Truffles

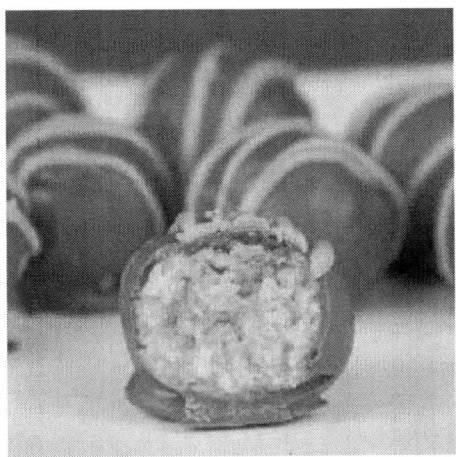

Ingredients:
5 tablespoons sunflower seed butter

1 tablespoon coconut oil
2 teaspoons vanilla extract
¾ cup almond flour
1 tablespoon flaxseed meal
pinch of low sodium salt
¼ cup sugar free dark chocolate chips
1 tablespoon cacao butter
chopped almonds (optional)
stevia to taste

Instructions:

1. Mix the ingredients in a bowl.
2. Using your hands mix until all ingredients are incorporated (I like using gloves when mixing so the oils from my skin do not get into the mixture)
3. Roll the dough into 1-inch balls and place them on a sheet of parchment paper and refrigerate for 30 minutes (using 2 teaspoons for each truffle will yield about 14 truffles)
4. Melt the chocolate chips in a double boiler along with the cacao butter
5. Dip each truffle in the melted chocolate, one at the time, and place them back on the pan with parchment paper
6. Top with chopped almonds and refrigerate until the chocolate is firm

Fetching Fudge

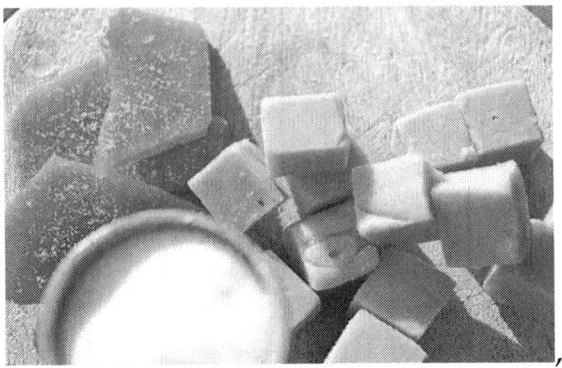

Ingredients:
1 cup coconut butter
1/4 cup coconut oil
1/4 cup cocoa
1/4 cup cocoa powder + 1 Tbsp
Stevia to taste
1 tsp vanilla

Instructions:
1. In the pot, gently melt the cocoa butter on low (number 2)
2. When it is half melted add the butter, the coconut oil and the coconut spread and gently mix with the whisk as it melts
3. Add vanilla, and stevia and whisk in well
4. Add the cocoa powder and whisk in well
5. Be sure to take the pot off the heat when the fat is melted and keep whisking until it is smooth and all the lumps are out — you don't want to overheat this Pour into the 8 x 8 pan that is lined with parchment paper
6. Refrigerate for 1 – 2 hours

7 When solid, pull the parchment paper out of the pan, put the block of fudge on a flat surface and cut into small squares

Enjoy! This will melt rather quickly — but it won't last long!

11) Conclusion

A really important aspect of reducing your inflammation is reducing your stress. If you are stressed out and worried about stuff, your body will not be able to help you heal. Adding stress and unrest to your life adds more distress. Studies show that people who are calm, relaxed, and less stressed tend to have better digestion and health. There are several methods of calming down and reducing stress that we will discuss here. Adjusting your diet alone might help you feel less stressed. If you are less worried about how you are feeling, you are going to end up adding more positivity to your life.

Stress is such a mean monster. It can wreak havoc on your internal system and how you take care of yourself. When you are stressed, it is easier to break and eat foods that you know you should not. When you eat these foods that cause inflammation in your body, your body sends you signals that makes you want to eat more of these foods that inflame your body. Take care of your body and your body will take care of you.

Finally, if you enjoyed this book, then I would like to ask you for a favor, would you be kind enough to leave a review for this book on Amazon? It would be greatly appreciated!

Thank you and good luck!

Made in the USA
Lexington, KY
10 December 2017